Handbook of Psychopharmacotherapy

A Life-Span Approach

Second Edition

Handbook of Psychopharmacotherapy

A Life-Span Approach

Second Edition

Mani N. Pavuluri, MD, PHD, FRANZCP
*Associate Professor of Psychiatry
Director, Pediatric Mood Disorders Clinic
and Bipolar Research Program
University of Illinois at Chicago*

Philip G. Janicak, MD
*Professor of Psychiatry
Medical Director, Psychiatric Clinical Research Center
Rush University
Chicago, Illinois*

Wolters Kluwer | Lippincott Williams & Wilkins
Health

Philadelphia · Baltimore · New York · London
Buenos Aires · Hong Kong · Sydney · Tokyo

Acquisitions Editor: Charles W. Mitchell *Production Editor:* Eve Malakoff-Klein
Managing Editor: Sirkka Howes Bertling *Designer:* Terry Mallon
Marketing Manager: Kimberly Schonberger *Compositor:* Aptara, Inc.

Second Edition

Library of Congress Cataloging-in-Publication Data

Pavuluri, Mani N.
    Handbook of psychopharmacotherapy: a life-span approach/Mani N.
    Pavuluri, Philip G. Janicak.—2nd ed.
        p. ; cm.
    Includes bibliographical references and index.
    ISBN-13: 978-0-7817-7196-2 (alk. paper)
    ISBN-10: 0-7817-7196-X (alk. paper)
    1. Psychopharmacology—Handbooks, manuals, etc. 2. Geriatric
psychopharmacology—Handbooks, manuals, etc. 3. Pediatric
psychopharmacology—Handbooks, manuals, etc. I. Janicak, Philip G.
II. Title.
    [DNLM: 1. Psychotropic Drugs—pharmacology—Handbooks. 2. Age
Factors—Handbooks. 3. Mental Disorders—drug therapy—Handbooks.
QV 39 P339h 2008]
    RM315.P37 2008
    615′.78—dc22
                                                    2007038031

Care has been taken to confirm the accuracy of the information present and to describe generally accepted practices. However, the authors, editors, and publisher are not responsible for errors or omissions or for any consequences from application of the information in this book and make no warranty, expressed or implied, with respect to the currency, completeness, or accuracy of the contents of the publication. Application of this information in a particular situation remains the professional responsibility of the practitioner; the clinical treatments described and recommended may not be considered absolute and universal recommendations.

    The authors, editors, and publisher have exerted every effort to ensure that drug selection and dosage set forth in this text are in accordance with the current recommendations and practice at the time of publication. However, in view of ongoing research, changes in government regulations, and the constant flow of information relating to drug therapy and drug reactions, the reader is urged to check the package insert for each drug for any change in indications and dosage and for added warnings and precautions. This is particularly important when the recommended agent is a new or infrequently employed drug.

    Some drugs and medical devices presented in this publication have Food and Drug Administration (FDA) clearance for limited use in restricted research settings. It is the responsibility of the health care provider to ascertain the FDA status of each drug or device planned for use in their clinical practice.

    To purchase additional copies of this book, call our customer service department at **(800) 638-3030** or fax orders to **(301) 223-2320**. International customers should call **(301) 223-2300**.

    Visit Lippincott Williams & Wilkins on the Internet: http://www.lww.com. Lippincott Williams & Wilkins customer service representatives are available from 8:30 am to 6:00 pm, EST.

10 9 8 7 6 5 4 3 2 1

Contents

Preface.. ix

1. First-generation Antipsychotics 1

2. Second-generation Antipsychotics 6
   Clozapine 6
   Risperidone 9
   Paliperidone Extended Release 11
   Olanzapine 13
   Olanzapine Plus Fluoxetne 14
   Quetiapine 15
   Ziprasidone 17
   Aripiprazole 21

3. First-generation Antidepressants 23

4. Second-generation Antidepressants 27
   Fluoxetine 27
   Sertraline 31
   Paroxetine 33
   Fluvoxamine 35
   Citalopram 37
   Escitalopram (S-CT) 39
   Venlafaxine 41
   Nefazodone 43
   Trazodone 45
   Mirtazapine 47
   Bupropion 49
   Duloxetine 51

5. Mood Stabilizers 53
   Lithium 53
   Valproate 57
   Lamotrigine 59
   Carbamazepine 61

6. Other Antiepileptic Agents 63
   Oxcarbazepine 63
   Gabapentin 65
   Tiagabine 67
   Topiramate 69
   Zonisamide 71

7. Anxiolytics/Sedative-Hypnotics 73
   Benzodiazepines 73
   Buspirone 77
   Pregabalin 79
   Zolpidem 81

Zaleplon 83
Eszoplicone 85
Ramelteon 87

8. Adjuvant Medications 89
    Clonidine 89
    Guanfacine 91

9. Psychostimulants 93
    Methylphenidate 93
    Concerta, Extended Release 95
    Methylphenidate Transdermal System 97
    Metadate Controlled Delivery 99
    Dexmethylphenidate 101
    Dextroamphetamine 103
    Adderall 105
    Modafinil 107
    Atomoxetine 109
    Lisdexamfetamine Dimesylate 111

10. Drug Therapy for Substance Use Disorders ... 116
    Naltrexone 116
    Naltrexone Extended Release 119
    Methadone 121
    Buprenorphine 123
    Disulfiram 125
    Acamprosate 127
    Varenicline 129

11. Cholinesterase Inhibitors and Related Drugs
    for the Elderly 131
    Donepezil 131
    Rivastigmine 133
    Galantamine 135
    Memantine 137

12. Miscellaneous Medications 139
    Propranolol 139
    Desmopressin 141

Appendices 143
    A Medication Clinic Progress Note Format .. 143
    B Lithium Laboratory Monitoring 144
    C Abnormal Involuntary Movement Scale—
       Modified (AIMS-M3D) 145
    D Pediatric Side Effects Checklist (P-SEC) .. 147
    E Abbreviations 151

Reference 155

Index 157

Preface

This book is for all clinicians, fellows, residents, and medical students who practice psychopharmacotherapy across the life span and need succinct and credible information to guide them in prescribing. It does not teach decision making about how to choose a drug for a specific disorder or symptom. Rather, it provides relevant information on a chosen drug. In addition, the book provides a quick reference about an agent's relative advantages and disadvantages in comparison to available alternatives. Information on drugs used to manage substance abuse, often not available in conventional textbooks, is also provided.

Although every attempt is made to be current, the reader must take into account that FDA-approved indications and preparations can change rapidly, with new drugs and formulations frequently being added to our current repertoire, as well as additional precautions and warnings. In summary, we offer information on available formulations, how to prescribe across the life-span, how to choose alternatives, and critical cautionary concerns.

For those seeking a more complete companion reference work, we would recommend *Principles and Practice of Psychopharmacotherapy,* 4th edition (Janicak et al., 2006).

We want to thank Naveen Reddy, MD, Soujanya Bogarapu, MD, and Ms. Sandra M. Smith for their invaluable help in the preparation of this handbook.

Mani N. Pavuluri and Philip G. Janicak

First-generation Antipsychotics

Mechanism of Action

Central dopamine receptor (e.g., D_2, D_3, and D_4) blockade. FGAs induce depolarization of dopamine neurons in nigrostriatal, mesolimbic, or other pathways (Table 1.1, Fig. 1.1).

Possible Advantage

Decreased dopaminergic activity improves certain symptoms of psychosis (e.g., positive symptoms).

Side Effects

Central Nervous System

- EPS: major side effect of FGAs; incidence of EPS is directly proportional to the potency of FGAs

  Acute EPS
  - Parkinsonian syndrome (occurs early in treatment and tends to persist if not treated)
  - Acute dystonia (occurs early in treatment and tends to persist if not treated)
  - Akathisia

  Late-onset (tardive) EPS: usually occurs after several months to years of drug exposure
  - Buccolinguomasticatory movements: sucking, smacking of lips
  - Choreoathetoid movements of tongue
  - Choreiform/athetoid movements of extremities and/or truncal areas
  - Any combination of these symptoms

- Sedation: inversely proportional to milligram potency. Usually occurs within a few days of treatment initiation (due to antihistamine action); can be avoided by shifting to a less sedating agent or giving the entire dose at bedtime
- Neuroleptic malignant syndrome: requires early recognition, immediate discontinuation of medication, supportive measures (e.g., cooling blankets), and other treatment (e.g., dantrolene)

Anticholinergic Effects

Blurred vision, dry mouth, constipation, urinary retention, cognitive disruption

Cardiovascular System

- Alpha-adrenergic blockade: orthostatic hypotension, reflex tachycardia
- Cardiac rhythm disturbances: prolongation of QT interval, torsade de pointes (especially thioridazine)

Table 1.1. Commonly used first-generation antipsychotics

Generic Name	Trade Name	Half-life (hr)	Dose Range (mg) per Day		Potency	Comments
			Adults	Children		
Chlorpromazine	Thorazine	24 (8–35)	100–1,000	Approved for children older than 6 mo	Low	• Sedation and ortho-static hypotension are common side effects.
			10–200	6 mo to 12 y: • Oral—0.25 mg/kg q.i.d. or b.i.d. • Rectal—1 mg/kg q.i.d. or t.i.d. • IM—0.5 mg/kg q.i.d. or t.i.d. Adolescents: 10 mg t.i.d. to 25 mg q.i.d.		• Photosensitivity, jaundice, and ocular deposits at higher doses are specific side effects.
Haloperidol	Haldol	24 (12–36)	3–30 0.25–4	Approved for children older than 3 y, 0.5–2 mg/d	High	• Significant EPS
Thioridazine	Mellaril	24 (6–40)	30–800 10–200	Approved for children older than 2 y 2–12 y: 0.5 mg/kg/d to a maximum of 3 mg/kg/d	Low	• Higher incidence of cardiac rhythm disturbances • Retinitis pigmentosa at doses >800 mg/d

				Older than 12 y: as in adults		• Delayed ejaculation; only used for treatment resistance or intolerance
Mesoridazine	Serentil	30 (24–48)	20–200 10–200	No information available	Low	• Available in parenteral form • Prolonged QT
Molindone	Moban	12 (6–24)	15–225 Elderly patients should be started on low dose.	Approved for children older than 12 y, 50–70 mg/d initial dose and increased to 100 mg/d in 3–4 d	Medium	• May cause less weight gain
Fluphenazine	Prolixin	18 (14–24)	5–40 0.25–4	Approved for children older than 12 y, 2.5–10 mg q.i.d. or t.i.d.	High	• Available in long-acting formulation
Trifluoperazine	Stelazine	18 (14–24)	2–30 1–15	Approved for children older than 6 y 6–12 y: 1 mg q.i.d. or b.i.d. Adolescents: 1–5 mg b.i.d.; optimal dose is 15–20 mg/d	High	—

(continued)

Table 1.1. (*Continued*)

Generic Name	Trade Name	Half-life (hr)	Dose Range (mg) per Day		Potency	Comments
			Adults	Children		
Thiothixene	Navane	34	6–40 1–15	Approved for children older than 12 y; no specific dose for children	High	—
Perphenazine	Trilafon	12 (8–21)	2–122–32	No information available	High	—
Loxapine	Loxitane	8 (3–12)	20–250 10–100	Approved for children older than 16 y; same as adults	Medium	—
Pimozide	Orap	55 (29–111)	1–10 0.25–4	Approved for children older than 12 y, 0.2 mg/kg/d; maximum, 10 mg/d	High	—

IM, intramuscular.

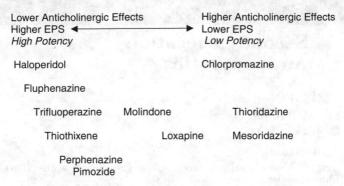

Figure 1.1.   First-generation antipsychotic side effects.

Endocrine Effects

- Decreased dopamine activity in the pituitary increases pro-lactin levels.
- May cause breast engorgement and lactation in women and gy-necomastia in men, as well as sexual dysfunction in both genders

Weight Gain

Less, particularly with high potency FGAs, compared with some second-generation antipsychotics

Drug Interactions

Avoid concomitant use with antacids, barbiturates, and lithium, which may decrease efficacy or increase toxicity.

Second-generation Antipsychotics

CLOZAPINE

Chemical Group
Dibenzodiazepine

Trade Name
Clozaril (Novartis Pharmaceuticals); generic clozapine (Ivax Pharmaceuticals, Inc.)

Forms Available
Clozaril caplets of 25 and 100 mg
Generic clozapine tablets of 12.5, 25, and 100 mg

Pharmacokinetics
Half-life is 5 to 15 hours, peaks in 1 to 4 hours, steady state in 3 to 4 days, bioavailability 60%

Dispensing
12.5 to 25 mg per day, then 25 mg b.i.d., increasing by 25 mg per day after reaching 100 mg. Dose is increased over a month. Wait long enough to assess for effects without increasing the dose. Taper carefully as cholinergic rebound/psychosis or other withdrawal symptoms including nausea, vomiting, diarrhea, and increased salivation may occur.

Range of Dosing
Adults: 25 to 900 mg per day
Children: Start at 12.5 mg once per day and gradually increase to no more than 3 to 6 mg per kg per day in divided doses.
Elderly: 10 to 100 mg per day

FDA Approval
Treatment-resistant schizophrenia; suicidal behavior in schizophrenia and schizoaffective disorder

Possible Mechanism of Action
Higher ratio of serotonin to dopamine antagonism: D_{1++}, D_2, D_3, D_{4+}, $5HT_{2c\,2a++}$

Possible Advantages
- Treatment-resistant psychosis, including schizophrenia, schizoaffective disorder, bipolar disorder
- May decrease suicidality in persons with schizophrenia and schizoaffective disorder (only agent with this FDA indication)
- Patients may continue to improve for 12 months or longer.
- EPS does not usually occur across recommended dosing range; decrease in tardive dyskinesia
- May improve negative symptoms (directly or indirectly)

Side Effects

- Agranulocytosis (see following section)
- Anticholinergic side effects
- Hypersalivation, especially nocturnal
- Tachycardia, low-grade fever, shorter corrected QTc interval (due to vagal inhibition)
- Weight gain: H_1 and $5HT_{2c}$ antagonism
- In the elderly population, may be too sedating; may produce anticholinergic and cardiovascular AEs; may also cause respiratory problems
- Seizures (1% to 2%): increased risk (3% to 5%) if dose is greater than or equal to 600 mg per day; may need to use anticonvulsant concomitantly, avoid carbamazepine
- Postural hypotension: α_1 antagonism
- Sedation: H_1 and α_1 antagonism (tolerance develops based on dose)
- Nocturnal enuresis
- Neuroleptic malignant syndrome
- Dyslipidemia
- Myocarditis
- New-onset diabetes; DKA

Agranulocytosis

Decrease in number of PMNL (i.e., absolute neutrophil count) less than 0.5% compared with 1% to 2%
  Idiosyncratic reaction, not dose related

Drug Interactions

Cimetidine, erythromycin, SSRIs, caffeine intake, smoking cessation, or risperidone may increase clozapine level.

Risk

Risk is less than 0.5% and other factors include:

- Time (95% of the cases in first 6 months, highest risk in first 4 to 18 weeks
- Sex (women have greater risk than men)
- Older age
- Ethnicity
- If increased/decreased WBC, increased ESR

Management[1]

- If WBC is less than 3,500 (or has dropped by a substantial amount from baseline), counts should be repeated.
- If WBC is less than 3,500 and/or the granulocyte count falls below 1,500, monitor twice weekly with differentials.
- If WBC is less than 3,000 and/or granulocyte count is less than 1,500, interrupt treatment and obtain CBC and differentials daily. May resume treatment if no symptoms of infection and WBC returns to greater than 3,000 plus greater than 1,500

[1]From Janicak PG, Davis JM, Perskorn SH, et al. *Principles and Practice of Psychopharmacotherapy.* 4th ed. Philadelphia: Lippincott Williams & Wilkins; 2006.

granulocyte count. Continue twice-weekly monitoring until WBC is greater than 3,500.
- If WBC is less than 2,000 or granulocytes is less than 1,000, stop clozapine and place the patient in reverse isolation with daily CBC and differential until levels return to normal. Do not rechallenge with clozapine.

Tests

For agranulocytosis, initially, draw CBC and differential count weekly; after 6 months, biweekly.

Plasma levels: 350 to 450 ng per mL for parent compound

RISPERIDONE

Chemical Group
Benzisoxazole

Trade Name
Risperdal (Janssen Pharmaceutica)
Risperdal Consta (Long-acting injectable formulation) (Janssen-Cilag)

Forms Available
Tablets of 0.25, 0.5, 1, 2, 3, and 4 mg; oral solution of 1 mg per mL in 100-mg bottle; m-TAB orally disintegrating tablets of 0.5, 1, and 2 mg
Risperidone microspheres 25, 37.5, and 50 mg IM

Pharmacokinetics
Half-life is 3 hours in fast metabolizers and 20 hours in poor metabolizers; half-life of its major metabolite 9-OH-risperidone is 21 to 30 hours; peaks in 1 to 3 hours; steady state in 1 to 5 days; bioavailability 70%.

Dispensing
Once a day is effective, but usually start as b.i.d. dose in adults and may continue as b.i.d. in children.

Range of Dosing
Adults: Usual range is 2 to 6 mg per day. Risperidone microspheres is usually given for adults 25 mg IM once every 2 weeks. Oral dose of 2 to 3 mg is given for the first 3 weeks. Maximum recommended dose is 50 mg IM.
Children: Start at 0.25 once a day or b.i.d. and gradually increase to 4 mg. Weight-based calculation is 0.1 to 0.5 mg per kg per day.
Elderly: 0.25 to 2 mg per day. May be activating, can cause EPS.

FDA Approval
Manifestations of psychotic disorders; bipolar mania and mixed episodes

Possible Mechanism of Action
Serotonin–dopamine (5-HT-DA) antagonism: $5HT_{2a}$ is greater than DA_2, preferentially distributed in frontal cortex and striatum. DA_2 antagonism reduces dopamine in prefrontal cortex; may improve positive symptoms; $5HT_2$ antagonism may improve negative and mood symptoms. No appreciable affinity for muscarinic cholinergic receptors.

Possible Advantages
- Improves positive symptoms
- Improves mood symptoms
- May decrease negative symptoms
- May decrease cognitive symptoms
- Fewer anticholinergic side effects
- Long-acting injectable formulation

Side Effects

- Increased risk of extrapyramidal symptoms, especially with dosages greater than 6 mg per day
- Postural hypotension: α_1 antagonism
- Increased prolactin: D_2 antagonism in tubero-infundibular tract
- Weight gain, sedation, decreased concentration
- 9-OH metabolite: QTc interval increased, clinical significance unknown
- Dyslipidemia
- New-onset diabetes; DKA
- Increased mortality in elderly patients with dementia-related psychosis

Pregnancy

Discontinue gradually 2 weeks before due date to avoid extrapyramidal symptoms in newborns. It is present in breast milk.

Drug Interactions

Metabolized by CYP 2D6; therefore, potentially subject to interactions with inhibitors such as fluoxetine, which may increase risperidone level

Tests

Check prolactin levels, if symptomatic. Lipid profile

PALIPERIDONE EXTENDED RELEASE

Chemical Group

Benzisoxazole derivative

Trade Name

Invega (Janssen Pharmaceutical)

Forms

Tablets of 3, 6, and 9 mg

Pharmacokinetics

Peak plasma concentration reached in 24 hours with an elimination half-life of 23 hours. Steady state is reached in 4 to 5 days.

Dispensing

Recommended dose is 6 mg once daily, administered in the morning. OROS® extended release provides a continuous release of medication over a 24-hour period, leading to minimal peaks and troughs in plasma concentrations. The OROS® drug release technology uses osmotic pressure to deliver at a controlled rate. The tablet consists of an osmotically active trilayer core composed of two drug layers containing the drug and excipients, and a push layer with the osmotically active components. Each tablet also has a water-dispersible overcoat, which in the GIT erodes quickly allowing water to enter the tablet through a semipermeable membrane that controls the rate at which water enters the tablet core. This process determines the rate of drug delivery. Patients should be informed that tablet residual may appear in stool.

Range of Dosing

Range is 3 to 12 mg per day.
Recommended initial and target dose is 6 mg once daily for adults, administered in the morning.

FDA Approval

Schizophrenia

Possible Mechanism of Action

Dopamine (D_2) and serotonin ($5HT_{2A}$) receptor antagonism

Possible Advantages

- Improves positive symptoms
- Improves mood symptoms
- May decrease negative symptoms
- May decrease cognitive symptoms
- Fewer anticholinergic side effects
- Less risk of hepatic drug–drug or drug–disease interactions
- Long-acting formulation in development

Side Effects

- Increased risk of extrapyramidal symptoms, especially with dosages greater than 6 mg per day
- Caution in patients with renal compromise
- Postural hypotension: α_1 antagonism

- Increased prolactin: D_2 antagonism in hypothalamic-pituitary tract
- Weight gain, sedation, decreased concentration
- 9-OH metabolite: QTc interval increased, clinical significance unknown
- New-onset diabetes; DKA
- Increased mortality in elderly patients with dementia-related psychosis

Contraindications
Hypersensitivity to paliperidone, risperidone, or any ingredients

Metabolism
CYP 2D6 and CYP 3A4 play a limited role in overall elimination. Pathways with a minor role in metabolism include dealkylation, hydroxylation, and dehydrogenation. The drug is primarily excreted in urine.

Drug Interactions
Levodopa and other dopamine agonists

Tests
Check prolactin levels, if symptomatic.
Lipid profile; plasma glucose; or HbA-1C

OLANZAPINE

Chemical Group

Thienobenzodiazepine

Trade Name

Zyprexa (Eli Lilly)

Forms Available

Tablets of 2.5, 5, 7.5, 10, 15, and 20 mg; Zydis orally disintegrating tablets of 5, 10, 15, and 20 mg, contains phenylalanine; IM injection of 10 mg

Pharmacokinetics

Half-life is 31 hours, peaks in 6 hours; steady state in 7 days; bioavailability 60%

Dispensing

Once a day dosing

Range of Dosing

Adults: usually 5 to 20 mg per day. Although the recommended maximum dose is 20 mg, this is often exceeded.

Children: 0.12 to 0.20 mg per kg body weight, given in 1 to 3 divided doses

Elderly: 2.5 to 10 mg per day

FDA Approval

Schizophrenia, bipolar mania, bipolar depression (combined with fluoxotine; see Olanzapine plus Fluoxetine, for more details)

Possible Mechanism of Action

Serotonin-dopamine antagonist: $5HT_2$; D_1, D_2, D_3, D_4

Possible Advantages

- Decreases positive symptoms
- Improves mood symptoms
- May decrease negative symptoms
- May improve cognitive symptoms
- No significant ECG changes

Side Effects

- D_2: increased prolactin (temporary, not sustained); akathisia may be seen with higher doses
- α_1: orthostatic hypotension, dizziness, and syncope
- M_1 to M_5: anticholinergic side effects
- H_1;$5HT_{2C}$: weight gain; somnolence
- New-onset diabetes; DKA
- Increased mortality in elderly patients with dementia and psychosis

Drug Interactions

- Benzodiazepines: orthostatic hypotension, syncope
- Carbamazepine, rifampin: lower olanzapine level
- Cimetidine, fluvoxamine, smoking cessation: increase olanzapine level

Tests

- Hepatic: increased SGPT
- Lipid profile
- Plasma glucose or HbA-1C

OLANZAPINE PLUS FLUOXETINE

Chemical Group

2-methyl-4-(4-methyl-1-piperazinyl)-10H-thieno[2,3-b][1,5]benzo-diazepine

Trade Name

Symbyax (Eli Lilly)

Forms Available

Capsules of olanzapine and fluoxetine hydrochloride (OFC) in four dosage options:

- Olanzapine 6 mg plus fluoxetine 25 mg
- Olanzapine 6 mg plus fluoxetine 50 mg
- Olanzapine 12 mg plus fluoxetine 25 mg
- Olanzapine 12 mg plus fluoxetine 50 mg

Dispensing

Usually taken once a day in the evening; may be taken with or without food

Range of Dosing

Adults: Should be administered once daily in the evening, generally beginning with the 6-mg/25-mg capsule. Although food has no appreciable effect on the absorption of olanzapine and fluoxetine given individually, the effect of food on its absorption has not been studied. Dosage adjustments, if indicated, can be made according to efficacy and tolerability. Antidepressant efficacy was demonstrated in a dose range of olanzapine 6 to 12 mg and fluoxetine 25 to 50 mg.

Children: no information available

Elderly: no information available

FDA Approval

Bipolar depression

Possible Mechanisms of Action

Same as those of olanzapine and fluoxetine

Mechanism of action is unknown, but it has been proposed that the monoaminergic neural systems (serotonin, dopamine, and norepinephrine) are responsible for enhanced antidepressant effect.

Possible Advantages

Using a single drug as mood stabilizer, offering the additional advantage of actively addressing depressive symptoms in bipolar disorder

Side Effects

Most common side effects are somnolence (22%), weight gain (21%), increased appetite (16%), and asthenia (15%).

Drug Interactions

Should not be used within 14 days of discontinuing MAOI. At least 5 weeks are allowed after stopping this agent before using MAOIs.

QUETIAPINE

Chemical Group
Dibenzothiazepine

Trade Name
Seroquel (AstraZeneca)
Seroquel XR (AstraZeneca)

Forms Available
Tablets of 25, 100, 200, and 300 mg
Extended release formulation tablets of 200, 300, and 400 mg

Pharmacokinetics
Half-life is 7 hours, peak in 1.5 hours; steady state in 2 days

Dispensing
On day 1, b.i.d. doses totaling 100 mg per day, increased to 400 mg per day on day 4 in increments of up to 100 mg per day in b.i.d. divided doses

Range of Dosing
Adults: 75 to 800 mg per day. Although the recommended maximum dose is 800 mg, this is often exceeded.
Children: Start at 12.5 or 25 mg once a day or b.i.d. and gradually increase to a maximum of 3 to 6 mg per kg per day in divided doses.
Elderly: 25 to 300 mg per day

FDA Approval
Schizophrenia; bipolar mania, bipolar depression

Possible Mechanism of Action
Serotonin-dopamine antagonism: $5HT_{2+++}$, $5HT_{6++}$, D_{1+}, D_{2+}, D_4. Some affinity for muscarinic cholinergic receptors.

Possible Advantages
- Decreases positive symptoms
- Improves mood symptoms
- May decrease negative symptoms
- May improve cognitive symptoms
- Extrapyramidal side effects are negligible across entire dosing range.
- Nonsustained prolactin elevation across entire dosing range
- No significant ECG changes

Side Effects
- α_1: orthostatic hypotension, dizziness, syncope
- H. antagonistic effects
- H_1: risk of somnolence higher during the 3 to 5 days of initial dose titration
- Transient increase in hepatic enzymes and decreases in total and free T_4
- Weight gain (usually moderate)

- Dyslipidemia
- New-onset diabetes; DKA
- Increased mortality in elderly patients with dementia and psychosis

Contraindications
Hypersensitivity

Metabolism
Metabolized by the liver; major metabolic pathways include sulfoxidation and oxidation

Drug Interactions
Metabolized by CYP 3A4, therefore potentially subject to interactions with ketoconazole and erythromycin, increasing quetiapine level. Thioridazine, phenytoin, and carbamazepine can decrease quetiapine level. Coadministration with divalproex increased plasma concentration.

Tests
Prescribing information recommends slit lamp eye examination at baseline and every 6 months with long-term treatment for persons at risk to develop cataracts. A causal relationship between cataract formation and quetiapine in humans has not been established.

ZIPRASIDONE

Chemical Group
Benzisothiazol

Trade Name
Geodon (Pfizer, Inc.)

Forms Available
Capsules of 20, 40, 60, and 80 mg
Injection (IM) of single-dose vial, 20 mg per mL, for acute parenteral use only

Pharmacokinetics
Half-life is 7 hours, peaks in 6 to 8 hours; steady state in 2 to 3 days; bioavailability increased twofold with food.

Dispensing
B.i.d. dosing

Range of Dosing

Adults: Efficacy was observed in dose ranges of 20 to 80 mg b.i.d. Maximum recommended dose is 160 mg but is often exceeded. Dose is increased after a minimum of 2 days.

Children: Start at 20 mg b.i.d. and gradually increase to no more than 40 mg b.i.d. Ziprasidone comes in capsules and cannot be administered at lower doses to preschool-age population. The optimal dosage in children has not been determined.

Elderly: There is no indication for reduced clearance of ziprasidone; however, due to multiple factors that may increase pharmacodynamic response or cause poorer tolerance or orthostasis, a lower starting dose and careful monitoring during the initial period should be considered.

FDA Approval
Schizophrenia and bipolar mania

Possible Mechanism of Action
Serotonin–dopamine antagonism: $5HT_{2a}$, $5HT_{1d}$, D_2 and D_3 antagonist, and $5HT_{1a}$ partial agonist. It is also an SSRI and a norepinephrine reuptake inhibitor. It has no appreciable affinity for muscarinic cholinergic receptors.

Possible Advantages
- Decreases positive symptoms
- Improves mood symptoms
- May decrease negative symptoms
- May improve cognitive symptoms
- No prolactin elevation
- Minimal risk of extrapyramidal symptoms
- May reverse weight gain and dyslipidemia

Side Effects
- Dose-related QTc prolongation (Fig. 2.1)

Maximum			Minimum

ACUTE EPS

←···→

Haloperidol	Risperidone	Olanzapine	Clozapine
	Paliperidone ER		Ziprasidone
	(Dose related)		Quetiapine
			Aripiprazole

PROLACTIN ELEVATION

←···→

Haloperidol	Ziprasidone	Clozapine
Risperidone		Quetiapine
Paliperidone ER	Olanzapine	Aripiprazole

QTc INTERVAL

←···→

Thioridazine	Ziprasidone	Risperidone
Mesoridazine	Paliperidone ER	Olanzapine
	Quetiapine	Haloperidol
		Aripiprazole

WEIGHT GAIN

←···→

Clozapine	Quetiapine	Ziprasidone
Olanzapine	Risperidone	Haloperidol
	Paliperidone ER	Aripiprazole

Figure 2.1.   Dose-related QTc prolongation. (Adapted from Janicak PG, Davis JM, Perskorn SH, et al. *Principles and Practice of Psychopharmacotherapy*. 4th ed. Philadelphia: Lippincott Williams & Wilkins; 2006.)

- Contraindicated in patients with known history of QT prolongation:
  - Congenital long QT syndrome
  - Recent acute myocardial infarction (MI) or uncompensated heart failure

  Risk is increased in patients with:
  - Bradycardia
  - Hypokalemia/hypomagnesemia
  - Concurrent drugs causing QT prolongation
- α_1 antagonism: postural hypotension, especially during initial dosing period
- Upper respiratory symptoms, sedation
- In pregnancy, discontinue gradually 2 weeks before due date to avoid extrapyramidal symptoms in newborns. Present in breast milk.

- New-onset diabetes; DKA (clinical and study results are favorable)
- Increased mortality in elderly patients with dementia and psychosis

Tests

Prescribing information recommends baseline K^+ and Mg^{2+} measurements. Baseline ECG in children (not an FDA requirement, but suggested in patients with potassium or sodium imbalance).

ARIPIPRAZOLE

Chemical Group

Quinolinone

Trade Name

Abilify (Bristol-Myers and Otsuka America Pharmaceuticals)

Forms Available

Tablets of 2, 5, 10, 15, 20, and 30 mg; DISCMELT orally disinte-grating tablets of 10, 15, 20, and 30 mg; oral as a 1 mg per mL solution; injection (IM) formulation in single dose vial 9.75 mg per 1.3 mL

Pharmacokinetics

Half-life is 75 hours; half-life of its major metabolite, dehydroarip-iprazole is 94 hours, peaks in 3 to 5 hours; steady state in 14 days; bioavailability 87%

Dispensing

Once a day, with or without food. However, due to possible nausea, administration with a meal is advised.

Range of Dosing

Adults: Recommended starting and target dose is 15 mg per day. Dose increase should be made after 2 to 3 weeks because this time frame is needed to achieve steady state.

Children: No information is available yet. Due to side effects such as nausea, it is recommended that aripiprazole be started at a lower dose (2.5 to 5 mg) and gradually increased.

Elderly: A lower starting dose is recommended because safety and efficacy have not been established in patients with psychosis associated with dementia.

FDA Approval

Schizophrenia, bipolar mania

Possible Mechanism of Action

Partial agonist at D_2 and $5HT_{1A}$ receptors and antagonist at postsynaptic $5HT_{2A}$ receptors. Partial agonist activity at D_2 and $5HT_{1A}$ is hypothesized to stabilize these neurotransmitter systems. Aripiprazole exhibits high affinity for D_2 (partial agonist), D_3, $5HT_{1A}$ (partial agonist), and $5HT_{2A}$ receptors. Moderate affinity for D_4, $5HT_{2c}$, $5HT_7$, α_1, and H_1 receptors; serotonin reuptake site. No appreciable affinity for muscarinic cholinergic receptors

Possible Advantages

- Decreases positive symptoms
- Improves mood symptoms
- May decrease negative symptoms
- May improve cognitive symptoms
- Minimal EPS
- No prolactin increase
- Minimal weight gain; may reverse dyslipidemia

- No clinically significant changes in hematology, serum chemistry, and urinalysis parameters
- No significant ECG changes

Side Effects

- Most common: headache (32%), nausea (14%), vomiting (12%), constipation (10%), anxiety (25%), insomnia (24%), dizziness (11%), akathisia (10%). EPS all types 6%, similar to placebo
- Dose-related side effect: somnolence
- Weight gain: Study data look favorable.
- New-onset diabetes; DKA (clinical and study results are favorable)
- Increased mortality in elderly patients with dementia and psychosis

Pregnancy

Caution: Safety in pregnancy is not established. Not recommended during breast feeding.

Metabolism and Drug Interaction

Aripiprazole is metabolized by biotransformation pathways: dehydrogenation (CYP 3A4 and CYP 2D6), hydroxylation, and N-dealkylation (CYP 3A4) by P450 enzymes.

Agents that induce CYP 3A4 (e.g., phenytoin, carbamazepine, rifampin) could cause increases in aripiprazole clearance, resulting in the need for higher doses. Inhibitors of CYP 3A4 (e.g., ketoconazole, fluoxetine, fluvoxamine) and CYP 2D6 (e.g., fluoxetine, paroxetine, quinidine) can inhibit aripiprazole elimination and cause increased blood levels. Dose should be adjusted accordingly.

3

First-generation Antidepressants

Chemical Group
HCAs
MAOIs

Trade Name
Refer to Table 3.1 for trade names.

Forms Available
- HCAs: tablets, capsules, and concentrates (see Table 3.1 for dose ranges)
- MAOIs:
  - Phenelzine, 15 mg tablet
  - Tranylcypromine, 10 mg tablet
  - Selegiline transdermal system (6, 9, or 12 mg per 24 hours) patch

Pharmacokinetics
HCAs

- Half-lives are usually 24 to 30 hours
- Therapeutic plasma levels include:

  Nortriptyline: 50 to 170 ng per mL
  Desimipramine: 110 to 160 ng per mL
  Amitriptyline: 80 to 150 ng per mL
  Imipramine: $\sim$250 ng per mL (threshold)

- Significant first-pass metabolism
- Substrates for CYP 2D6, CYP 3A3/4
- Highly protein bound
- Highly lipophilic

MAOIs

- Half-lives are short (i.e., 2 to 4 hours), but half-life of MAO inhibition is $\sim$2 weeks because it takes that period to synthesize the new enzyme.
- Undergo "first-pass" degradation, so alterations in metabolism (genetic, acquired) could affect bioavailability and/or efficacy
- Patch formulation at 6 mg per 24 hours avoids tyramine–drug interaction by avoiding inhibition of MAO-A in GIT.

Dispensing
Initially, b.i.d. until optimal dose is determined and acclimation to side effects is achieved. Then usually can administer once daily. If higher doses (e.g., 250 to 300 mg per day) are required, may need to give b.i.d. to minimize side effects. Selegiline TS is administered in patch formulation (6, 9, or 12 mg per 24 hours).

Range of Dosing
Refer to Table 3.1 for dose ranges.

Table 3.1. First-generation antidepressants

Drug	Trade Name	Dose Range (mg/d)
Heterocyclics		
Amitriptyline	Elavil	75–300
Imipramine	Tofranil	75–300
Doxepin	Sinequan	75–300
Desipramine	Norpramin	75–300
Nortriptyline	Pamelor	75–300
Trimipramine	Surmontil	75–200
Protriptyline	Vivactil	20–60
Clomipramine	Anafranil	100–250
Maprotiline	Ludiomil	75–225
Dibenzoxazepine		
Amoxapine	Ascendin	200–600
Phenylpiperazine		
Trazodone	Desyrel	150–600
Monoamine oxidase inhibitors		
Phenelzine	Nardil	15–90
Tranylcypromine	Parnate	30–60
Selegiline TS	Emsam	6–12 mg/24 hr patch

FDA Approval
- HCAs: depression, OCD (clomipramine)
- MAOIs: depression; atypical depression

Possible Mechanism of Action
- NE and 5HT reuptake inhibition
- MAO-A, MAO-B
  - Nonselective (A **and** B) or selective (A **or** B)
  - Irreversible or reversible
- HCAs
  - Downregulation of NE and 5HT receptors
- MAOIs
  - Inhibit degradation of NE, DA, and 5HT
  - Irreversible inhibition of MAO by covalently bonding to the enzyme (e.g., phenelzine, tranylcypromine)
  - Newer agents may be selective for MAO-A (e.g., clorgyline) or MAO-B (e.g., l-deprenyl) and reversibly inhibit the enzyme (e.g., moclobemide).

Anatomic sites of action
- Locus coeruleus
- Raphe nuclei

Possible Advantages
HCAs may be more effective for severe depression, whereas MAOIs may be more effective for atypical depression.

Table 3.2. Side effects of first-generation antidepressants

Drugs	Sedation	Anticholinergic	Orthostatic Hypotension	Cardiac Effects
Heterocyclics				
Amitriptyline	High	High	Moderate	High
Clomipramine	High	High	Low	Moderate
Desipramine	Low	Low	Low	Moderate
Doxepin	High	Moderate	Moderate	Moderate
Imipramine	Moderate	Moderate	High	High
Maprotiline	Moderate	Moderate	Low	Moderate
Nortriptyline	Moderate	Moderate	Low	Moderate
Protriptyline	Low	Moderate	Low	Moderate
Trimipramine	High	High	Moderate	High
Dibenzoxazepines				
Amoxapine*	Low	Low	None	None
Phenylpiperazine				
Trazodone	High	Low	Moderate	Low
Monoamine oxidase inhibitors				
Phenelzine	Low	Low	High	None
Tranylcypromine	High	Very low	Very low	None
Selegiline TS	Low	Low	Low	None

*May cause extrapyramidal symptoms (EPS) due to active metabolite effects.

Side Effects

For adverse effects, refer to Table 3.2; cardiac arrhythmias are most serious and potentially lethal.

Possible increase in suicidal ideation or behavior in pediatric group and young adults up to age 24.

- Black box warning
- Not FDA approved in pediatric population

Drug Interactions

- HCAs: CYP 2D6 substrates, so metabolism will be altered by inhibitors or inducers of this isoenzyme
- MAOIs: May cause hypertensive crisis with high-tyramine-content foods or with certain medications (e.g., pseudoephedrine) and life-threatening 5HT syndrome when combined with other potent 5HT agents (e.g., SSRIs)

4

Second-generation Antidepressants

FLUOXETINE

Chemical Group
(+/−)-N-methyl-3-phenyl-3-[α, α, α-trifluoro-p-tolyl)-oxy] propylamine hydrochloride

Trade Name
Prozac (Eli Lilly); generic fluoxetine (Barr Labs)

Forms Available
Prozac: capsules of 10, 20, and 40 mg; tablets of 10 mg; elixir 20 mg per 5 mL (mint flavored); long-acting form (Prozac Weekly) available as 90-mg capsule, with a booster pack of four tablets for a month's supply.
   Generic fluoxetine: tablets and capsules of 10, 20, and 40 mg; elixir 20 mg per 5 mL

Pharmacokinetics
Half-life is 1 to 3 days for fluoxetine (increases to 4 to 6 days with chronic administration); 7 to 9 days for norfluoxetine. Prozac Weekly is the delayed-release form given once a week. It consists of enteric coated pellets released in the small bowel. Peak concentration in blood is the same as that of the 20-mg tablet, but troughs and steady-state concentrations are lower than those of the IR tablets given once daily. Plasma concentrations may not be predictive of clinical response.

Dispensing
Once a day. Long-acting form starts to release medication in 10 hours. When making the transition from IR to long-acting form, need a week's overlap with both medications. Separate the first 90-mg weekly dose and the last 20-mg once-daily dose by 1 week.

FDA Approval
Depression, OCD, bulimia nervosa, panic disorder, PMDD
Only SSRI approved for depression in pediatric population

Possible Mechanism of Action
Inhibition of 5HT reuptake transport mechanism

Range of Dosing
Adults: starting dose is 20 mg; maximum of 80 mg per day. Wait 4 weeks to increase the dose.
Children: start at 5 to 10 mg if anxious (20 mg for teenagers) once a day and gradually increase to a maximum of 0.25 to 1 mg per kg per day.

Elderly: 5 to 40 mg per day. An upper dose range has not been established for the elderly; may be activating and cause insomnia; long half-life.

OCD: higher maintenance dose, response in 12 to 26 weeks

Panic disorder: starting dose must be very low; maintenance dose is higher. Target symptoms may first worsen; usually more than 50% improvement in symptoms is eventually observed.

Bulimia: higher starting dose, higher maintenance dose; effect in 3 to 8 weeks.

Site of Action

Serotonin reuptake transporter

Possible Mechanism of Action

- Pre- and postsynaptic receptors are upregulated secondary to depletion of 5HT.
- With SSRI, 5HT is increased in somatodendritic area, then downregulates $5HT_{1A}$ autoreceptors.
- More 5HT is released.
- Downregulation of serotonin post- and presynaptic receptors then occurs.

Anatomical Sites of Action in CNS and Indications/Actions

- Midbrain raphe–frontal lobe: depression
- Basal ganglia: OCD
- Hippocampus: panic disorder
- Hypothalamus: bulimia
- Spinal cord: pain

Possible Advantages

No adverse cardiovascular effects, wide therapeutic index

Side Effects

- $5HT_2$: agitation, akathisia, anxiety, panic, insomnia; subsides over time
- $5HT_3$: diarrhea, GI distress, and nausea (particularly high with Prozac Weekly)
- CNS: headache
- Sexual dysfunction: due to dopamine lowering and 5HT increase in mesolimbic area and at the level of ANS; possibly mediated by $5HT_2$; lower dose or switch to mirtazapine, bupropion, or nefazodone
- Possible long-term side effects: apathy; sexual dysfunction (do not increase the dose if secondary to depression)

Warning: Antidepressants increased the risk of suicidal thinking and behavior (suicidality) in short-term studies in children, adolescents, and young adults in short-term studies of MDD and other psychiatric disorders. Anyone considering the use of fluoxetine or any other antidepressant in a child or adolescent must balance this risk with the clinical need. Short-term studies did not show an increase in the risk of suicidality with antidepressants compared to placebo in adults beyond age 24; there was a reduction in risk with antidepressants compared to placebo in adults aged 65 and older. Depression and certain other psychiatric disorders are associated with increases in the risk of suicide. Patients of all ages who are started on antidepressant therapy should be monitored appropriately and observed closely for clinical worsening, suicidality, or unusual changes in behavior. Families and caregivers should be advised of the need for close observation and communication with the prescriber. Fluoxetine is approved for use in pediatric patients with MDD and OCD.

Drug Interactions

- Inhibits CYP 2D6—may elevate plasma levels of pimozide, phenytoin, CBZ, desipramine, imipramine, amitriptyline, nortriptyline, and certain antiarrhythmics
- Stop at least 5 weeks before starting an MAOI or thioridazine.

SERTRALINE

Chemical Group
(1S-cis)-4-(3,4-dichlorophenyl)-1,2,3,4-tetrahydro-N-methyl-1-nanphthalenamine hydrochloride

Trade Name
Zoloft (Pfizer); generic sertraline (Ivax/Teva); generic sertraline oral concentrate (Roxane)

Forms Available
Tablets of 25, 50, and 100 mg; syrup also available, but tastes bad
Generic sertraline: tablets of 25, 50, and 100 mg; oral concentrate 20 mg per mL

Pharmacokinetics
Half-life is 25 hours, metabolites 60 to 70 hours allowing for easier withdrawal

Dispensing
Once a day

Range of Dosing
Adults: 25 to 200 mg per day
Children: start at 25 mg once a day and gradually increase to no more than 100 mg for 4 to 6 weeks, then increase the dose further if necessary and if tolerated. Usually, give no more than 1.5 to 3 mg per kg per day.
Elderly: 12.5 to 150 mg per day. Can cause nausea and GI upset; may be sedating

FDA Approval
Depression, OCD (adults and children), PTSD, panic disorder, and PMDD

Possible Mechanism of Action
Inhibition of 5HT reuptake transport mechanism

Possible Advantages
- Once a day dosing
- Fewer withdrawal symptoms
- Possibly less activating than fluoxetine
- Fewer anticholinergic side effects

Side Effects
- As in all SSRIs
- $5HT_3$ effect greater than in the periphery: more diarrhea compared with others
- Can cause agitation, akathisia

Warning: Antidepressants increased the risk of suicidal thinking and behavior (suicidality) in short-term studies in children, adolescents, and young adults in short-term studies of MDD and other psychiatric disorders. Anyone considering the use of sertraline or any other antidepressant in a child or adolescent must balance this risk with the clinical need. Short-term studies did not show an increase in the risk of suicidality with antidepressants compared to placebo in adults beyond age 24; there was a reduction in risk with antidepressants compared to placebo in adults aged 65 and older. Depression and certain other psychiatric disorders are associated with increases in the risk of suicide. Patients of all ages who are started on antidepressant therapy should be monitored appropriately and observed closely for clinical worsening, suicidality, or unusual changes in behavior. Families and caregivers should be advised of the need for close observation and communication with the prescriber. Sertraline is not approved for use in pediatric patients except for patients with OCD.

Drug Interactions

- Inhibits CYP 2D6; contraindicated for use with pimozide due to potential elevation of pimozide levels; may also increase levels of desipramine, imipramine, amitriptyline, nortriptyline, and certain antiarrhythmics.
- Stop at least 2 weeks before starting an MAOI or thioridazine.

PAROXETINE

Chemical Group
Phenylpiperidine-salt

Trade Name
Paxil (Smith Kline, Beecham); generic paroxetine (Apotex)

Forms Available
Tablets of 10, 20, 30, and 40 mg
CR tablets (Paxil CR): 12.5, 25, and 37.5 mg
Orange-flavored suspension: 10 mg per 5 mL in 250-mL bottles
Generic paroxetine: tablets of 10, 20, 30, and 40 mg; oral suspension 10 mg per 5 mL

Pharmacokinetics
Half-life is 24 hours for IR form and 15 to 20 hours for CR form. No active metabolites; therefore, poses a greater risk for withdrawal symptoms.

Dispensing
Once a day. CR form has a degradable polymeric matrix designed to control dissolution rate of paroxetine over ~4 to 5 hours. Also, enteric coated CR form delays start of release until tablet exits the stomach.

Range of Dosing

IR form
Adults: 10 to 60 mg per day
Children: start at 10 to 20 mg once a day. Do not exceed 0.25 to 0.70 mg per kg per day.
Elderly: 5 to 40 mg per day.

CR form
Adults: recommended initial dose is 2 mg (CR) per day for MDD and 12.5 mg for panic disorder. If not responding, increase dose in 12.5-mg increments at intervals of at least 1 week. Maximum dose should not exceed 62.5 mg for MDD and 75 mg for panic disorder.
Children: no information available yet.
Elderly: recommended initial dose is 12.5 mg per day, may be increased if necessary, not to exceed 50 mg per day.

FDA Approval
IR form: major depression, OCD, panic disorder, social anxiety disorder, GAD, PTSD
CR form: major depression, panic disorder

Possible Mechanism of Action
Inhibition of 5HT reuptake transport mechanism

Possible Advantages
Anxiety mixed with depression

Side Effects

- As in all SSRIs
- Mild anticholinergic effects
- Not good for patients with sleep difficulties

Warning: Antidepressants increased the risk of suicidal thinking and behavior (suicidality) in short-term studies in children,
adolescents, and young adults in short-term studies of MDD
and other psychiatric disorders. Anyone considering the use of
Paroxetine or any other antidepressant in a child or adolescent must balance this risk with the clinical need. Short-term
studies did not show an increase in the risk of suicidality with
antidepressants compared to placebo in adults beyond age 24;
there was a reduction in risk with antidepressants compared
to placebo in adults aged 65 and older. Depression and certain other psychiatric disorders are associated with increases
in the risk of suicide. Patients of all ages who are started on
antidepressant therapy should be monitored appropriately and
observed closely for clinical worsening, suicidality, or unusual
changes in behavior. Families and caregivers should be advised
of the need for close observation and communication with the
prescriber. Paroxetine is not approved for use in pediatric patients.

Patients currently taking paroxetine should not be discontinued abruptly, due to risk of discontinuation symptoms. At the
time that a medical decision is made to discontinue an SSRI or
other newer anti-depressant drug, a gradual reduction in the
dose rather than an abrupt cessation is recommended.

Drug Interactions

- Potent inhibitor of CYP 2D6; therefore, may increase levels of
  pimozide, desipramine, imipramine, amitriptyline, nortriptyline, and certain antiarrhythmics; may also inhibit its own
  metabolism
- Also metabolized by CYP 2D6; therefore, levels may be increased by cimetidine and decreased by phenobarbital and
  phenytoin
- In case of serious hepatic and renal problems, use lower doses
  with maximum dose not more than 50 mg per day.
- Requires at least a 2-week washout before starting an MAOI or
  thioridazine

FLUVOXAMINE

Chemical Group
2-aminoethyl oxime ether of aralkylketone

Trade Name
Luvox (Solvay Pharmaceuticals); generic fluvoxamine (Eon Labs)

Forms Available
Tablets of 25, 50, and 100 mg
Generic fluvoxamine: tablets of 25, 50, and 100 mg

Pharmacokinetics
Half-life 15 hours; steady state in 1 week; bioavailability is 50% and unaffected by food.

Dispensing
B.i.d.

Range of Dosing
Adults: 150 to 300 mg per day
Children: start at 25 mg b.i.d. or 50 mg once a day and increase to a tolerable and effective dose, given b.i.d. Do not exceed 1.5 to 4.5 mg per kg per day or 200 mg per day in children.
Elderly: 50 to 150 mg per day.

FDA Approval
OCD

Possible Mechanism of Action
Inhibition of 5HT reuptake transport mechanism

Possible Advantages
Anxiety mixed with depression

Side Effects
• As in all SSRIs
• Nausea and vomiting may be higher than with other SSRIs

Warning: Antidepressants increased the risk of suicidal think-ing and behavior (suicidality) in short-term studies in children, adolescents, and young adults in short-term studies of MDD and other psychiatric disorders. Anyone considering the use of fluvoxamine or any other antidepressant in a child or adoles-cent must balance this risk with the clinical need. Short-term studies did not show an increase in the risk of suicidality with antidepressants compared to placebo in adults beyond age 24; there was a reduction in risk with antidepressants compared to placebo in adults aged 65 and older. Depression and cer-tain other psychiatric disorders are associated with increases in the risk of suicide. Patients of all ages who are started on antidepressant therapy should be monitored appropriately and observed closely for clinical worsening, suicidality, or unusual changes in behavior. Families and caregivers should be advised of the need for close observation and communication with the prescriber. Fluvoxamine is not approved for use in pediatric patients except for patients with OCD.

Drug Interactions
- Inhibits CYP 1A2; therefore, may increase levels of theophylline (decrease dose), warfarin, and propranolol
- Inhibits CYP 3A4; therefore, contraindicated with pimozide and may increase levels of alprazolam and diazepam
- Requires at least a 2-week washout before starting an MAOI or thioridazine

CITALOPRAM

Chemical Group
A racemic, bicyclic phthalane derivative

Trade Name
Celexa (Forest Pharmaceuticals); generic citalopram (Alpharma Inc.)

Forms Available
Tablets of 10, 20, and 40 mg; peppermint solution 10 mg per 5 mL
Generic citalopram: tablets of 10, 20, and 40 mg; oral solution 10 mg per 5 mL

Pharmacokinetics
Half-life is 35 hours; steady state in 1 week; bioavailability is 80% and unaffected by food.

Dispensing
Once a day

Range of Dosing
Adults: 10 to 60 mg per day.
Children: start at 10 to 20 mg once a day. Do not exceed 0.25 to 0.70 mg per kg per day.
Elderly: recommended dose is 20 mg per day.

FDA Approval
Depression

Possible Mechanism of Action
Inhibition of 5HT reuptake transport mechanism

Possible Advantages
Most selective SSRI; often preferred if there are multiple medical problems due to minimal drug interactions involving the CYP 450 enzyme system

Side Effects
• As in all SSRIs
• Possibly fewer sexual side effects

Warning: Antidepressants increased the risk of suicidal thinking and behavior (suicidality) in short-term studies in children,
adolescents, and young adults in short-term studies of MDD
and other psychiatric disorders. Anyone considering the use of
Citalopram or any other antidepressant in a child or adolescent must balance this risk with the clinical need. Short-term
studies did not show an increase in the risk of suicidality with
antidepressants compared to placebo in adults beyond age 24;
there was a reduction in risk with antidepressants compared
to placebo in adults aged 65 and older. Depression and certain other psychiatric disorders are associated with increases
in the risk of suicide. Patients of all ages who are started on
antidepressant therapy should be monitored appropriately and
observed closely for clinical worsening, suicidality, or unusual

changes in behavior. Families and caregivers should be advised of the need for close observation and communication with the prescriber. Citalopram is not approved for use in pediatric patients.

Drug Interactions
- Weak inhibitor of CYP 2D6
- Requires at least a 2-week washout before starting an MAOI or thioridazine

ESCITALOPRAM (S-CT)

Chemical Group
Phthalane derivative

Trade Name
Lexapro (Forest Pharmaceuticals); generic escitalopram (Ivax)

Forms Available
Tablets of 5, 10, and 20 mg or as an oral solution of 1 mg per mL
Generic escitalopram: tablets of 5, 10, and 20 mg

Pharmacokinetics
Half-life 27 to 30 hours; steady state in 1 week; bioavailability is 80% and unaffected by food.

Dispensing
Once a day, with or without food (pending study); 10 and 20 mg of escitalopram is bioequivalent to 20 and 40 mg of citalopram, respectively.

Range of Dosing
Adults: recommended starting and maintenance dose is 10 mg
Children: no specific guidelines available yet
Elderly: 10 mg per day for most elderly patients; however, escitalopram should be used with caution in elderly patients with decreased hepatic, renal, or cardiac function, coexistence of other diseases, as well as concomitant drug therapy

FDA Approval
MDD, GAD

Possible Mechanism of Action
Highly potent blockade of serotonin reuptake transport mechanism S-CT without its inactive R-enantiomer

Possible Advantages
- No significant reuptake inhibition of NE or D
- Low affinity for serotonin, adrenergic, histamine, muscarinic, and BZD receptors
- Minimal drug interactions involving the CYP 450 enzyme system
- Reported faster onset of action and greater overall magnitude of effect than citalopram

Side Effects
Same as with citalopram: nausea, diarrhea, insomnia, dry mouth; possibly fewer sexual side effects

Warning: Antidepressants increased the risk of suicidal thinking and behavior (suicidality) in short-term studies in children, adolescents, and young adults in short-term studies of MDD and other psychiatric disorders. Anyone considering the use of escitalopram or any other antidepressant in a child or adolescent must balance this risk with the clinical need. Short-term studies did not show an increase in the risk of suicidality with antidepressants compared to placebo in adults beyond age 24; there was a reduction in risk with antidepressants compared to placebo in adults aged 65 and older. Depression and certain other psychiatric disorders are associated with increases in the risk of suicide. Patients of all ages who are started on antidepressant therapy should be monitored appropriately and observed closely for clinical worsening, suicidality, or unusual changes in behavior. Families and caregivers should be advised of the need for close observation and communication with the prescriber. Escitalopram is not approved for use in pediatric patients.

Drug Interactions
S-didesmethyl-CT, a metabolite of S-CT, is a moderate inhibitor of CYP 2C9 and 2C19. Contraindicated with MAOIs. Needs caution when used with antimigraine medications.

VENLAFAXINE

Chemical Group
Phenethylamine bicyclic derivative

Trade Name
Effexor (Wyeth Ayerst); generic venlafaxine (Teva)

Forms Available
Tablets of 25, 37.5, 50, 75, and 100 mg; XR in 37.5-, 75-, and 150-mg capsules.
Generic venlafaxine: tablets of 25, 37.5, 50, 75, and 100 mg

Pharmacokinetics
Half-life 5 hours; metabolite 11 hours; steady state in 3 days

Dispensing
B.i.d.; XR available for once-daily use.

Range of Dosing
Adults: 75 to 225 mg in XR form, up to 375 mg in regular form
Children: start at 25 to 37.5 mg b.i.d. Do not exceed 1 to 3 mg per kg per day.
Elderly: no dose adjustment is recommended. As with any drug for the treatment of depression or GAD, however, caution should be used when treating the elderly, especially when increasing the dose.

FDA Approval
Depression; GAD

Possible Mechanism of Action
Serotonin and norepinephrine reuptake inhibitor (SNRI) $\pm$ Dopamine reuptake inhibitor (DRI)
Low dose: primarily SRI (one: serotonin)
Medium dose: SRI + norepinephrine reuptake inhibitor (NRI) (two: serotonin, noradrenaline)
High dose: SNRI + dopamine and adrenergic reuptake inhibitor (DARI) (three: serotonin, noradrenaline, dopamine)

Possible Advantages
- Depression refractory to other agents; melancholia
- Decreased problems with weight gain, hypersomnia; may benefit atypical depression
- Reported more rapid onset of action with higher initial dose, if tolerated
- No A_1, H_1, or M_1 side effects

Side Effects
- Treatment-emergent anxiety
- At higher doses, may increase blood pressure; use in hypertensive and anxious patients should be more carefully monitored
- Headache
- Insomnia

- Sweating
- Weight loss in first 5 months and then possible weight gain

Withdrawal symptoms may be seen with sudden cessation (e.g., GI effects, dizziness, sweating).

Warning: Antidepressants increased the risk of suicidal thinking and behavior (suicidality) in short-term studies in children, adolescents, and young adults in short-term studies of MDD and other psychiatric disorders. Anyone considering the use of venlafaxine or any other antidepressant in a child or adolescent must balance this risk with the clinical need. Short-term studies did not show an increase in the risk of suicidality with antidepressants compared to placebo in adults beyond age 24; there was a reduction in risk with antidepressants compared to placebo in adults aged 65 and older. Depression and certain other psychiatric disorders are associated with increases in the risk of suicide. Patients of all ages who are started on antidepressant therapy should be monitored appropriately and observed closely for clinical worsening, suicidality, or unusual changes in behavior. Families and caregivers should be advised of the need for close observation and communication with the prescriber. Venlafaxine is not approved for use in pediatric patients.

Metabolism and Drug Interactions
- CYP 2D6 inhibitor
- 14-day washout prior to an MAOI or thioridazine

4. Second-generation Antidepressants 43

NEFAZODONE

Chemical Group
Phenylpiperazine

Trade Name
Generic nefazodone (Mylan, Ranbaxy, Teva, and Watson)

Forms Available
Generic nefazodone: tablets of 50, 100, 150, 200, and 250 mg
Serzone brand has been removed from the market and is no longer available.

Pharmacokinetics
Half-life is 2 to 4 hours; longer in elderly.

Dispensing
B.i.d. in adults; once a day is adequate in the elderly.

Range of Dosing
Adults: 200 to 600 mg; usually greater than or equal to 300 mg
per day is most efficacious
Children: 1 to 8 mg per kg per day
Elderly: 50 to 200 mg per day; upper dose range not established

FDA Approval
Depression, GAD

Possible Mechanism of Action
$5HT_2$ antagonist + serotonin receptor antagonist and reuptake inhibitor (SARI)

Possible Advantages
Due to $5HT_2$ receptor antagonism:
- Decreased anxiety
- Increased slow-wave sleep
- Decreased sexual dysfunction

Side Effects
- A_1 antagonism-counteracted norepinephrine reuptake inhibitor (NRI) = no orthostatic hypotension
- Sedation
- Hepatic toxicity and failure

Warning: Antidepressants increased the risk of suicidal thinking and behavior (suicidality) in short-term studies in children, adolescents, and young adults in short-term studies of MDD and other psychiatric disorders. Anyone considering the use of nefazodone or any other antidepressant in a child or adolescent must balance this risk with the clinical need. Short-term studies did not show an increase in the risk of suicidality with antidepressants compared to placebo in adults beyond age 24; there was a reduction in risk with antidepressants compared to placebo in adults aged 65 and older. Depression and certain other psychiatric disorders are associated with increases in the risk of suicide. Patients of all ages who are started on antidepressant therapy should be monitored appropriately and observed closely for clinical worsening, suicidality, or unusual changes in behavior. Families and caregivers should be advised of the need for close observation and communication with the prescriber. Nefazodone is not approved for use in pediatric patients.

Ordinarily, treatment with nefazodone should not be initiated in individuals with active liver disease or with elevated baseline serum transaminases levels. There is no evidence that pre-existing liver disease increases the likelihood of developing liver failure; however, baseline abnormalities can complicate patient monitoring.

Patients should be alert for signs and symptoms of liver dysfunction (e.g., jaundice, anorexia, GI complaints, malaise) and to report them to their doctor immediately.

Metabolism and Drug Interactions

- CYP 3A4; metabolite formed (MCPP/5HT$_{2AC}$ agonist)
- Four percent of whites have no 2D6 to inhibit MCPP; so stimulate with opposite effect on 5HT$_{2AC}$. Diagnosis suspected if there are flulike symptoms at onset. Palinopsia secondary to partial agonism of 5HT$_2$.
- Contraindicated with pimozide and CBZ
- Inhibitor of CYP 3A4; therefore, may increase levels of triazolam, alprazolam, statins, cyclosporine, and tacrolimus.

TRAZODONE

Chemical Group
Triazolopyridine derivative

Trade Name
Desyrel (Apothecon); generic trazodone/Trazalon (Barr, Pliva, Teva, Watson, Mutual/URL)

Forms Available
Tablets of 50, 100, 150, and 300 mg
Generic trazodone: tablets of 50, 100, 150, and 300 mg

Pharmacokinetics
Half-life is 10 to 15 hours; bioavailability increased with food.

Dispensing
Once-a-day if less than or equal to 100 mg

Range of Dosing
Adults: 150 to 400 mg per day
Children: there is no recommended dose available. In clinical practice, starting dose is 25 mg q.h.s. It may be increased to 50 mg for sleep difficulties.
Elderly: 25 to 200 mg per day

FDA Approval
Depression

Possible Mechanism of Action
$5HT_2$ antagonism + SRI

Possible Advantages
Has been used in lower doses to manage sleep difficulties (it does not interfere with REM sleep pattern)

Side Effects
- Priapism
- A_1 antagonism/orthostatic hypotension
- H_1 antagonism: sedation

Warning: Antidepressants increase the risk of suicidal thinking and behavior (suicidality) in short-term studies in children, adolescents, and young adults in short-term studies of MDD and other psychiatric disorders. Anyone considering the use of trazodone or any other antidepressant in a child or adolescent must balance this risk with the clinical need. Short-term studies did not show an increase in the risk of suicidality with antidepressants compared to placebo in adults beyond age 24; there was a reduction in risk with antidepressants compared to placebo in adults aged 65 and older. Depression and certain other psychiatric disorders are associated with increases in the risk of suicide. Patients of all ages who are started on antidepressant therapy should be monitored appropriately and observed closely for clinical worsening, suicidality, or unusual changes in behavior. Families and caregivers should be advised of the need for close observation and communication with the prescriber. Trazodone is not approved for use in pediatric patients.

Drug Interactions
- May increase levels of digoxin and phenytoin
- Amprenavir and cimetidine may increase levels of trazodone.

MIRTAZAPINE

Chemical Group
Piperazino-azepine group

Trade Name
Remeron (Organon); generic mirtazapine (Mylan, Teva, Prasco)

Forms Available
Tablets of 15, 30, and 45 mg
Generic mirtazapine: tablets of 15, 30, and 45 mg

Pharmacokinetics
Half-life is 20 to 40 hours; bioavailability is 80% and unaffected
by food.

Dispensing
Once daily

Range of Dosing
Adults: up to 45 mg per day
Children: optimal dose is not known.
Elderly: 7.5 to 45 mg per day

FDA Approval
Depression

Possible Mechanism of Action
Noradrenaline and specific serotonergic antidepressant (NaSSA):
increases NE; increases $5HT_{1A}$ receptor stimulation; antagonizes
$5HT_2$ and $5HT_3$ receptors

Possible Advantages
• Refractory depression/SSRI nonresponders; HIV patients, to
  improve appetite; anorexia nervosa; weight gain; anxious depression; no interference with sexual function; no nausea or
  diarrhea
• Overall, $5HT_2$ and $5HT_3$ receptor antagonism improves tolerability of this drug.

Side Effects
H_1 antagonism causes weight gain and sedation, but also may
contribute to reduction in anxiety.

Warning: Antidepressants increased the risk of suicidal thinking and behavior (suicidality) in short-term studies in children,
  adolescents, and young adults in short-term studies of MDD
  and other psychiatric disorders. Anyone considering the use of
  mirtazapine tablets or any other antidepressant in a child or
  adolescent must balance this risk with the clinical need. Short-
  term studies did not show an increase in the risk of suicidality with antidepressants compared to placebo in adults beyond
  age 24; there was a reduction in risk with antidepressants
  compared to placebo in adults aged 65 and older. Depression

and certain other psychiatric disorders are associated with increases in the risk of suicide. Patients of all ages who are started on antidepressant therapy should be monitored appropriately and observed closely for clinical worsening, suicidality, or unusual changes in behavior. Families and caregivers should be advised of the need for close observation and communication with the prescriber. Mirtazapine is not approved for use in pediatric patients.

Drug Interactions

Metabolized by CYP 3A4; therefore, decreased levels may occur when coprescribed with protease inhibitors, ketoconazole, erythromycin, nefazodone, and cimetidine

BUPROPION

Chemical Group
Aminoketone group

Trade Name
Wellbutrin; Zyban (Glaxo Wellcome); Wellbutrin XL (Anchen Pharmaceuticals) generic bupropion (Sun, Teva, IMPAX)

Forms Available
IR formulation available in 75- and 100-mg tablets; SR formulation available in 100, 150, and 200 mg
Generic bupropion: tablets of 75, 150, and 300 mg; XL tablets of 150 and 300 mg

Pharmacokinetics
Half-life 14 hours

Dispensing
B.i.d., unless XL is used

Range of Dosing
Adults: 100 mg first day, 200 to 300 mg by fourth day, effect seen in 2 to 4 weeks
Children: starting dose is 100 mg per day, increased up to 150 mg SR, if necessary. This dose is maintained unless the child weighs more than 150 lb.
Elderly: 75 to 225 mg per day. May be activating.

FDA Approval
Depression; smoking cessation (Zyban)

Possible Mechanism of Action
NRI + DRI

Possible Advantages
• Psychomotor retardation
• Atypical depression with excess sleepiness
• Pseudodementia
• May be less likely to induce switch to mania or rapid cycling in bipolar disorder
• Less sexual dysfunction
• No orthostatic hypotension or cardiac problems
• Used for smoking cessation
• May be used for stimulant withdrawal/craving
• Used as second-line drug in ADHD

Side Effects
• Risk of seizure increases with doses greater than 150 mg per day or 450 mg per day IR and greater than 200 mg per day or 400 mg per day SR
• Contraindicated in patients with an eating disorder or seizure disorder due to increased seizure risk

Warning: Although Zyban is not indicated for treatment of depression, it has the same active ingredient as antidepressant medications containing bupropion (e.g., Wellbutrin, Wellbutrin SR, and Wellbutrin XL). Antidepressants increased the risk of suicidal thinking and behavior (suicidality) in short-term studies in children, adolescents, and young adults in short-term studies of MDD and other psychiatric disorders. Anyone considering the use of bupropion or any other antidepressant in a child or adolescent must balance this risk with the clinical need. Short-term studies did not show an increase in the risk of suicidality with antidepressants compared to placebo in adults beyond age 24; there was a reduction in risk with antidepressants compared to placebo in adults aged 65 and older. Depression and certain other psychiatric disorders are associated with increases in the risk of suicide. Patients of all ages who are started on antidepressant therapy should be monitored appropriately and observed closely for clinical worsening, suicidality, or unusual changes in behavior. Families and caregivers should be advised of the need for close observation and communication with the prescriber. Bupropion is not approved for use in pediatric patients.

Drug Interactions

• Inhibits CYP 2B6 and CYP 2D6; therefore, may increase levels of pimozide, desipramine, imipramine, amitriptyline, nortriptyline, and certain antiarrhythmics
• 14-day washout with an MAOI

DULOXETINE

Chemical Group
Thiophenepropylamine hydrochloride

Trade Name
Cymbalta (Eli Lilly and Co.)

Forms Available
Capsules of 20-, 30-, and 60-mg strengths
   Delayed-release capsules are available in 20-, 30-, and 60-mg strengths

Pharmacokinetics
Half-life ~12 hours (range 8 to 17 hours)

Dispensing
20 mg b.i.d. with increases at intervals of no less than 1 week, 40-mg dose increments; target dose of 60 mg b.i.d.

Range of Dosing
Adults: 40 to 120 mg per day
Children: little experience with using this medication
Elderly: little experience with using this medication

FDA Approval
• MDD
• Neuropathic pain
• GAD
• Fibromyalgia (pending)

Possible Mechanism of Action
Potent and relatively balanced inhibition of the 5HT and NE reuptake transporters; weak inhibitor of DA reuptake transporter

Possible Advantages
• Lacks significant affinity for muscarinic, histaminergic, α-adrenergic, dopaminergic, serotonergic, and opioid receptors
• May produce greater efficacy than agents acting on a single neurotransmitter system
• May benefit painful physical symptoms associated with depression
• Does not appear to cause significant elevation in blood pressure

Side Effects
• Nausea
• Headache
• Dry mouth
• Constipation
• Sweating
• Fatigue
• Insomnia/somnolence

Warning: Antidepressants increased the risk of suicidal thinking and behavior (suicidality) in short-term studies in children, adolescents, and young adults in short-term studies of MDD and other psychiatric disorders. Anyone considering the use of duloxetine or any other antidepressant in a child or adolescent must balance this risk with the clinical need. Short-term studies did not show an increase in the risk of suicidality with antidepressants compared to placebo in adults beyond age 24; there was a reduction in risk with antidepressants compared to placebo in adults aged 65 and older. Depression and certain other psychiatric disorders are associated with increases in the risk of suicide. Patients of all ages who are started on antidepressant therapy should be monitored appropriately and observed closely for clinical worsening, suicidality, or unusual changes in behavior. Families and caregivers should be advised of the need for close observation and communication with the prescriber. Duloxetine is not approved for use in pediatric patients.

Contraindications
Hypersensitivity, MAOIs, uncontrolled narrow-angle glaucoma

Metabolism
Elimination of duloxetine is mainly through hepatic metabolism involving two P450 isozymes, CYP2D6 and CYP1A2. Most (~70%) of the duloxetine dose appears in the urine as metabolites of duloxetine; ~20% is excreted in the feces.

Pregnancy
No data available

Drug Interactions
- Duloxetine is both an inhibitor and substrate of CYP P450 2D6
- MAOIs

Tests
No specific laboratory tests are required.

Mood Stabilizers

LITHIUM

Chemical Group
Monovalent cation

Trade Names and Available Forms
- Eskalith capsule—300 mg (Smith Kline, Beecham)
- Eskalith CR tablets—450 mg (Smith Kline, Beecham)
- Lithobid SR tablets—300 mg (Solvay Pharmaceuticals, Inc.)
- Lithium citrate syrup—8 mEq per mL = 300 mg (Solvay Pharmaceuticals, Inc.)
- Lithium carbonate capsules—150, 300, and 600 mg

Pharmacokinetics
Half-life is 24 hours; steady state in 5 days; reaches peak level in 2 hours with regular formulation, 4 hours with SR forms

Dispensing
Start as t.i.d. dosing; can be given once a day after reaching a steady-state therapeutic level.

Range of Dosing
Adults: 300 mg b.i.d. or t.i.d. in adults. Start slow, increase by 300 mg every 1 to 3 days. Therapeutic level is 0.5 to 1.5 mEq per L.
Children: 10 to 30 mg per kg per day; usually begin with IR once a day 150 or 300 mg; gradually increase to a therapeutic level of 0.6 to 0.8 mEq per L and reassess.
Elderly: 75 to 1500 mg per day. Elderly patients often require lower lithium dosages to achieve therapeutic serum levels. They may also exhibit adverse reactions at serum levels ordinarily tolerated by younger patients. Drug may cause cognitive side effects resembling dementia.

FDA Approval
Bipolar disorder: acute mania, maintenance

Possible Mechanism of Action
Modifying second messenger system:
- Blocks recycling of inositol phosphate from PIP_2
- Inhibits adenylate cyclase enzyme (generates cAMP), which alters G-protein interaction with neurotransmitters. This mechanism may also be responsible for side effects via pancreas, thyroid, and kidney.

Possible Advantages
- Prophylaxis to prevent recurrence (0.8 to 1.0 mEq per L)
- Moderate effect for acute treatment and prophylaxis of recurrent depressive episode
- Violence, personality disorder with mood instability: trial for 12 weeks at 0.6 to 1.2 mEq per L

- May decrease suicide risk in bipolar disorder
- May have neuroprotective effect

Side Effects

- Early, as level is rising:
  - Nausea, tremor
  - SR provides excellent bioavailability with fewer peak-level side effects, but has a tendency to cause diarrhea due to slower absorption in small bowel.
- Common: thirst, urination, weight gain, tremor, dermatological/acne
- GI side effects: nausea, vomiting, anorexia, diarrhea, abdominal pain (citrate syrup may lessen these symptoms).

Withdrawal Effects

Prudent to decrease by 300 mg every 2 to 4 weeks; abrupt discontinuation (less than or equal to 2 weeks) may precipitate mood episode.

RENAL.

- Tubulointerstitial nephritis may occur.
- Long-term effects are seen in persons who take divided doses versus once-a-day doses; only slight increase in sclerotic glomeruli/atrophic tubules
- Polyuria: anti-ADH action; in the long term, 50% to 70% are affected. Ten percent develop nephrogenic diabetes and produce more than 3 L of urine per day. These symptoms usually improve with dosage reduction or discontinuation; rarely, may need permanent treatment with K^+ sparing diuretic or amiloride.
- Nephrotic syndrome: should not be given lithium again

NEUROLOGIC.

- 7- to 16-Hz tremor similar to essential tremor, increased by anxiety; propranolol may help
- Benign intracranial hypertension (due to poor absorption of cerebrospinal fluid, diagnosis by fundoscopy), causing headache

COGNITIVE.   Dulling effect, slowing

THYROID.

- Inhibits TSH-responsive adenyl cyclase
- Interferes with thyroid hormones at multiple sites: iodine uptake, tyrosine iodination, release of T_3/T_4
- Timing of onset is variable.

PARATHYROID.

- Can cause hypoparathyroidism (uncommon)

CARDIAC.

- Benign: T-wave flattening
- Serious: SA block; tachycardia; clinical features include syncope and palpitation
- May require ECG monitoring

DERMATOLOGIC.

- Acne, psoriasis, folliculitis–pruritus–hyperkeratitis

GENERAL.
- Hair loss
- Weight gain: 10 kg in 20% of patients (possibly due to insulinlike effect)
- Blood: benign increase in WBC

Toxicity

The degree of toxicity can be classified as:

- Early signs—ataxia, dysarthria, lack of coordination
- Mild—occurs in the range of 1.5 to 2.0 mEq per L; most often characterized by listlessness, nausea, slurring of speech, diarrhea, and coarse tremors
- Moderate—occurs in the range of 2.0 to 2.5 mEq per L; most often characterized by coarse tremors and other CNS symptoms such as confusion or delirium, pronounced ataxia
- Severe—begins with levels at 2.5 to 3.0 mEq per L; most often characterized by significant alterations in consciousness, spontaneous attacks of hyperextension of extremities, choreoathetosis, seizures, coma, or death

With an acute overdose, treatment includes the use of various supportive measures because no antidote is available. The initial recommended steps are:

- Serum measurement of lithium, creatinine, electrolytes, and plasma osmolality
- Gastric lavage
- Monitoring of fluid intake and output
- Obtaining a history about the timing and amount of lithium taken
- Neurological examination including mental status examination and baseline EEG

Special Groups

Rapid cyclers: not as initially responsive, but may show improvement over a longer time period
Elderly: start 300 mg b.i.d. only; GFR is decreased
Pregnancy: GFR increased; may need higher levels. At parturition, there is risk of toxicity due to loss of water; Ebstein's anomaly in newborns exposed to lithium in the first trimester
Children: dysarthria, nocturnal enuresis

Metabolism and Drug Interactions

- Thiazides are absorbed at the renal distal convoluted tubule. Sodium and lithium are reabsorbed at the renal proximal convoluted tubule and loop only, so thiazides will increase lithium levels by 30% to 50%.
- NSAIDs and ACE inhibitors can increase lithium level.
- Coffee and theophylline can decrease lithium level.

Tests

- Serum level 12 hours after last dose: after 5 to 7 days with each dose change; when level is stable, check every 6 to 12 months

- RFT: 24-hour pretreatment creatinine clearance; BUN and serum creatinine every 6 to 12 months
- TFT every 6 to 12 months
- Electrolytes every 6 to 12 months
- Serum HCG in women of child-bearing age
- Screening ECG

VALPROATE

Chemical Group

2-Propyl-pentanoic acid

Trade Name

Depacon, Depakote, Depakene (Abbott Laboratories)

Forms Available

- Divalproex[1] sodium delayed-release (DR) tablets (Depakote): 125, 250, and 500 mg
- Divalproex sodium ER tablets (Depakote): 250 and 500 mg
- Divalproex sodium-coated particles in capsules (Depakote Sprinkles): 125 mg
- Valproic acid (Depakene): 250 mg capsule and 250 mg per 5 mL syrup
- Sodium valproate (Depacon) (injectable): 500 mg per 5 mL

Pharmacokinetics

Half-life is 8 hours for the DR tablets and 9 to 16 hours for the ER preparations.

Dispensing

Usually b.i.d

Range of Dosing

Adults: 250 mg t.i.d. or full-dose rapid titration with 15 to 30 mg per kg body weight; check for side effects; adequate serum levels achieved in 2 to 3 days. Final level can be at 50 to 150 μg per mL. Depakote ER is administered as a single dose. The ER form is not bioequivalent to the DR tablets given b.i.d. because they cause 20% less fluctuation in concentration. If dosage adjustment is required in smaller doses than the ER form, then the DR forms must be used. Recommended dose for ER is 500 mg once daily for a week and then increasing to 1,000 mg once daily the next week based on tolerability and need.

Children: 15 to 20 mg per kg per day

Elderly: 125 to 1,800 mg per day. May cause weight gain and impair concentration and recall.

FDA Approval

Bipolar disorder, acute mania; seizure disorders

- Depakene: approved for monotherapy or adjunctive therapy for simple and complex absence seizures and adjunctive therapy for patients with multiple seizures, including absence seizures
- Depakote: approved for monotherapy and adjunctive therapy for complex partial seizures alone or in association with other disorders; also as monotherapy for bipolar mania
- Depacon: approved for same indications as Depakene and Depakote when injectable form is indicated

Possible Mechanism of Action

- Increases GABA at BDZ site
- Opens chloride channel

[1] Divalproex = sodium valproate + valproic acid.

- Synergistic action with lithium
- Inhibits PKC

Possible Advantages
- Epilepsy and mood problems
- Acute mania
- Prophylaxis for mania, depression; mixed and rapid cycling episodes may be resistant to lithium
- Cyclothymia at very low doses (125 to 500 mg per day)
- Affective disorders in developmentally disabled persons
- PTSD
- Migraine
- Panic disorder
- May have neuroprotective effects

Side Effects
- Hepatotoxicity; thrombocytopenia; pancreatitis (idiosyncratic)
- Rash
- Weight gain, increased appetite
- Hair loss
- GI distress—nausea, vomiting, and diarrhea (less with divalproex)
- Cognitive dulling
- Pregnancy—neural tube defects (~1%)
- Possibly contributes to PCOS
- Most serious adverse effects: hepatic failure (primarily in the very young), pancreatitis, and teratogenicity (black box warnings)

Metabolism and Drug Interactions
- In children younger than 2 years, metabolites cause hepatic impairment.
- Salicylates increase valproic acid level.
- Lamotrigine level is doubled by valproic acid.
- SSRIs and valproic acid mutually increase each other's levels.
- Rifampin and anticonvulsants may increase valproate levels.

Tests
- CBC: check for leukopenia, thrombocytopenia
- LFT: hepatic transaminase increase
- Pancreatic enzymes

LAMOTRIGINE

Chemical Group
Phenyltriazine

Trade Name
Lamictal (Glaxo Wellcome)

Forms Available
Tablets of 25, 100, 150, and 200 mg; chewable/dispersible tablets of 25 mg

Pharmacokinetics
Half-life ~15 hours; varies depending on age and use of concomitant anticonvulsants

Dispensing
B.i.d.; when stopping, should be withdrawn over 2 weeks

Range of Dosing
Adults: 300 to 500 mg per day; gradual dosing (25-mg increments) to prevent rash
Children: 2 to 10 mg per kg per day. Refer to prescribing information for doses when initiating therapy; usually dosed by weekly increments of 25 (in the first 4 weeks at least) to 50 mg (post 4 weeks, in adolescents) to decrease risk of rash.
Elderly: Dose selection for the elderly should be cautious, usually starting at the low end of the dosing range.

FDA Approval
- Monotherapy for bipolar disorder, maintenance phase
- Adjunctive therapy in adults with partial seizures; in pediatric and adult patients, for generalized seizures in Lennox–Gastaut syndrome
- Monotherapy in adults with partial seizures

Possible Mechanism of Action
Inhibition of voltage-sensitive sodium channels, which stabilize neuronal membranes and modulate presynaptic release of excitatory transmitters (e.g., glutamate, aspartate). Also, there is possible weak inhibition of serotonin $5HT_3$ receptors.

Possible Advantages
- Alternative choice for stabilizing mood
- May have acute antidepressant and antimanic effects
- Bipolar II, rapid cyclers

Side Effects
- Blood: WBC will usually fall if dose is increased faster than 100 mg per week; pure red cell aplasia
- Dermatologic: in 10% of cases; rash occurs within 4 to 6 weeks, maculopapular-erythematous eruptions; less than 1% may develop more serious Stevens–Johnson syndrome or toxic epidermal necrolysis (angioedema, lymphadenopathy)
- Accumulates in melanin-containing tissues

- Hepatic failure
- GI: nausea, vomiting, diarrhea
- Neurologic: somnolence, dizziness, ataxia, tremor, headache, diplopia, blurred vision

Metabolism and Drug Interactions

All the AEDs decrease lamotrigine level except valproate, which increases levels; therefore, dose should be decreased when combined with valproate.

CARBAMAZEPINE

Chemical Group
5H-dibenzapine-5-carboxamide

Trade Name
Equetro (Shire); Tegretol (Novartis Pharmaceuticals)

Forms Available
Equetro: ER capsules of 100, 200, and 300 mg
Tegretol: tablets of 200 mg; chewable tablets of 100 mg; liquid
(syrup) 100 mg per 5 mL; Carbatrol ER sprinkles 200- and
300-mg capsules

Pharmacokinetics
Half-life 18 to 55 hours; due to autoinduction may fall to 5 to 20
hours with repeated dosing, plateaus in 3 to 5 weeks; peak levels
in 4 to 8 hours

Dispensing
Tegretol: b.i.d. or t.i.d
Equetro: b.i.d

Range of Dosing
Adults: 4 to 12 μg per mL, core range 6 to 10 μg per mL. Start with
200 mg b.i.d., increasing by 200-mg increments to 1,000 mg
per day. Can do more rapid titration in 2 weeks. Recommended
maximum dose of 1,800 mg. Check for autoinduction in 2 to
6 weeks. For Equetro: Recommended initial dose is 400 mg per
day given in divided doses, b.i.d. Dose should be adjusted in
200-mg daily increments to achieve optimal clinical response.
Maximum dose is 1,600 mg per day.
Children: 10 to 30 mg per kg day. Start at a low dose of 200 mg
QHS or 200 mg b.i.d., and increase depending on the tolerability (within 1 week to 1 month) to reach therapeutic level.
Safety and effectiveness of Equetro in pediatric and adolescent
patients have not been established.
Elderly: 50 to 1,200 mg per day. Can cause agranulocytosis

FDA Approval
- ER formulation is approved for bipolar disorder, acute mania
(Equetro)
- Seizure disorder (Tegretol)
  - Partial seizure with complex symptomatology
  - Generalized tonic-clonic seizures
  - Mixed seizure patterns
- Trigeminal neuralgia (Tegretol)

Possible Mechanism of Action
Inhibits repetitive firing of action potentials by inactivating Na^+
channels. Inhibits kindling (i.e., repeated subthreshold activity
that can produce epileptic activity)

Possible Advantages

Helpful in rapid cycling; takes 6 to 12 months to judge. May not decrease all affective recurrences. Helpful in acute mania, neuropathic pain, impulse control, and alcohol withdrawal

Side Effects

- Rapid dose increase: nausea, vomiting, slurred speech, dizziness, drowsiness, ataxia
- Dose related: sedation, low WBC, high LFT, ataxia, cognitive slowing (motor more than mental)
- Less dose related: tremor, cardiac conduction delay, SIADH-hyponatremia, low T_3/T_4
- Idiosyncratic: rash 10 days after (red, raised, itchy), rarely severe
- Hepatitis
- Blood dyscrasias: aplastic anemia, low WBC (less than 4,000), low platelets (less than 100,000), bone marrow toxicity

Toxicity/Overdose

(Due to rapid increase in levels): nystagmus, tremor, respiratory depression; Treatment: supportive; hemodialysis not effective because highly protein bound

Pregnancy

Craniofacial defects (11%), developmental delay, neural tube defects (~1%)

Metabolism and Drug Interactions

Potent inducer of P450 system; includes autoinduction; SSRIs can inhibit CBZ metabolism.

Tests

CBC with platelets every 6 to 12 months; stop if WBC is less than 3,000, neutrophils less than 1,500;

- LFT, RFT, and TFT every 6 to 12 months.

Other Antiepileptic Agents

OXCARBAZEPINE

Chemical Name

10, 11-Dihydro-10-oxo-5-H dibenzazepine-5 carboxamide

Trade Name

Trileptal (Novartis Pharmaceuticals)

Forms Available

Tablets of 150, 300, and 600 mg; 60 mg per mL oral suspension

Pharmacokinetics

Half-life for parent compound: 2 hours; for active metabolite: 9 hours; reaches peak serum concentration in 2 to 3 days

Dispensing

B.i.d.

Range of Dosing

Adults: initial dose is 300 mg b.i.d.; usual daily dose is 1,200 mg per day in two divided doses. Dosage increases are made every 3 days in increments of 150 or 300 mg, depending on weight and tolerability.

Children: 8 mg per kg per day and should not exceed 600 mg per day given in two divided doses

Elderly: start at lowest possible dose. Clinical trials have shown that oxcarbazepine in elderly patients produced maximum plasma concentrations and area under the curve (AUC) values of 10-monohydroxy-derivative (MHD) that are 30% to 60% higher than in younger patients. Age-related creatinine clearance is the cause.

FDA Approval

Adults: monotherapy or adjuvant therapy for partial seizure disorder

Children: adjuvant therapy for partial seizure disorder, ages 4 to 16 years

Possible Mechanism of Action

Results from parent compound, as well as MHD. MHD blocks voltage-sensitive sodium channels, stabilizing hyperexcited neuronal membranes, inhibiting repetitive firing, and decreasing the propagation of synaptic impulses. These actions are believed to prevent seizures or rage attacks and aggression.

Possible Advantages

- Rapid cycling; takes 6 to 12 months to judge
- May not decrease all affective recurrences
- May be helpful in acute mania, neuropathic pain, disorders of impulse control, alcohol withdrawal

Side Effects

- No dose adjustment is needed for hepatically impaired subjects.
- There is a linear correlation between creatinine clearance and renal clearance of MHD.
- Rapid dose increase may cause headache, nausea, vomiting, slurred speech, dizziness, drowsiness, and ataxia.
- Dose related: low sodium levels, ataxia, cognitive slowing (motor more than mental)
- Treatment of overdose: supportive; hemodialysis is not helpful because 40% of MHD is protein bound.

Metabolism and Drug Interactions

Completely absorbed and extensively metabolized to MHD. It can inhibit CYP 2C19 and induce CYP 3A4/5.

Tests

CBC; leukocytopenia, thrombocytopenia); electrolytes (low potassium and sodium); serum creatinine; LFT; GGT, serum transaminases elevated.

GABAPENTIN

Chemical Group
1-(Aminomethyl) cyclohexaneacetic acid

Trade Name
Neurontin (Parke-Davis); generic gabapentin (Teva, Alpharma)

Forms Available
Capsules of 100, 300, and 400 mg; tablets of 600 and 800 mg; oral solution 250 mg per 5 mL
   Generic gabapentin: capsules of 100, 300, and 400 mg; tablets of 600 and 800 mg

Pharmacokinetics
Half-life 5 to 9 hours, peaks in 2 to 3 hours, reaches steady state in 1 to 2 days

Dispensing
T.i.d.

Range of Dosing
Adults: start at 300 mg per day, then 300 mg b.i.d. on second day, then 300 mg t.i.d. on third day; 1,800 mg per day for epilepsy and 900 to 1,500 mg per day for mood disorders in adults. Range is 200 to 3,600 mg per day.
Children: 5 to 30 mg per kg per day.
Elderly: more likely to have decreased renal function. Care should be taken in dose selection based on creatinine clearance values in these patients:

- Creatinine clearance greater than 60 mL per min = 400 mg t.i.d.
- Creatinine clearance greater than 30 to 60 mL per min = 300 mg t.i.d.
- Creatinine clearance greater than 15 to 30 mL per min = 300 mg q.i.d.

FDA Approval
Adjunctive therapy of partial seizures with and without secondary generalization in adults with epilepsy and for postherpetic neuralgia

Possible Mechanism of Action
Structurally similar to GABA, but does not act through GABA receptors. Its action is undefined, and studies show that it has possible affinity for cholinergic receptors in the neurons of the brain but not in the periphery. Possibly increases GABA in the substantia nigra as well.

Possible Advantages
- Has a lipophilic cyclohexane ring that allows it to cross blood–brain barrier; increases GABA only in substantia nigra–increased synthesis and accumulation of GABA
- Decreased release of DA, NE, 5HT

- Binding site is calcium channel subunit
- Wide therapeutic index, so blood levels are unnecessary
- Anxiolytic effect; doubtful mood-stabilizing effect
- Neuropathic pain and migraine

Side Effects
- Common: somnolence, dizziness, ataxia, fatigue
- Uncommon:
  - lowers WBC, platelets
  - weight gain
  - stuttering
  - involuntary twitches
  - hypomania
- In pregnant rats: hydronephrosis and hydroureters

Metabolism and Drug Interactions
No drug interactions; eliminated by kidneys; cimetidine decreases renal clearance

TIAGABINE

Chemical Group
(−)-(R)-1-[4,4-Bis(3-methyl-2-thienyl)-3- butenyl] nipecotic acid hydrochloride

Trade Name
Gabitril (Cephalon); Gabitril (Abbott Laboratories)

Forms Available
Tablets: 2, 4, 6, 8, 10, 12, and 16 mg

Pharmacokinetics
The elimination half-life is 7 to 9 hours, with peak plasma concentrations occurring at ~ 45 minutes following an oral dose; hence it is taken with food for slower absorption. The pharmacokinetics of tiagabine are linear over the single dose range of 2 to 24 mg; after multiple dosing, steady state is achieved within 2 days.

Dispensing
B.i.d. to q.i.d.

Range of Dosing
Adults: start at 4 mg per day, then increase weekly by 4 to 8 mg per day until clinical response or up to 56 mg per day.
Children: used only in children 12 years or older, dose range is 4 to 32 mg per day
Elderly: not known

FDA Approval
Adjunctive therapy of partial seizures in adults and children 12 years and older

Possible Mechanism of Action
Blocks sodium channels and also enhances GABA receptors

Possible Advantages
• Potential role in treatment of refractory bipolar mood disorder
• Adjunctive therapy for inadequately controlled partial epilepsy

Side Effects
• Common: dizziness, somnolence, depression, confusion, asthenia
• Uncommon: serious skin rash; EEG abnormalities and status epilepticus reported

Metabolism and Drug Interactions
CBZ and phenytoin decrease tiagabine levels. Tiagabine decreases valproate levels. No interaction with cimetidine.

TOPIRAMATE

Chemical Group
Sulfamate-substituted monosaccharide

Trade Name
Topamax (Ortho-McNeil Neurologics, Inc.)

Forms Available
Tablets of 25, 100, and 200 mg; sprinkle capsules of 15 and 25 mg

Pharmacokinetics
Half-life less than or equal to 15 hours

Dispensing
B.i.d.

Range of Dosing
Adults: start at 50 mg per day. Increase to 400 mg per day in divided doses. Discontinue gradually.
Children: 3 to 6 mg per kg per day. For very young children, start at 25 mg per day and increase by 25 mg every other day.
Elderly: In clinical trials, no age-related difference in effectiveness or adverse reactions was seen. The possibility of age-associated renal functional abnormalities should be considered.

FDA Approval
Adjunctive therapy (in adults) of partial onset seizures, primary generalized tonic-clonic seizures, Lennox–Gastaut syndrome, prophylaxis of migraines, monotherapy epilepsy in patients 10 years of age and older

Possible Mechanism of Action
Blocks sodium channels and also enhances GABA receptors

Possible Advantages
Weight loss; questionable mood stabilizing and anxiolytic effects

Side Effects
• Cognitive dulling
• Confusion and memory problems
• Parethesias
• Kidney stones
• Acute myopia and secondary angle closure glaucoma
• Unknown effect in pregnancy

Metabolism and Drug Interaction
CBZ decreases topiramate levels; oral contraceptives less effective; with valproic acid, mutual decrease in levels; can be used in older patients; children metabolize rapidly

ZONISAMIDE

Chemical Group
Sulfonamide; 1–2-benzisoxazole-3-methanesulfonamide

Trade Name
Zonegran (Elan Pharmaceuticals)

Forms Available
Capsule of 100 mg

Pharmacokinetics
Half-life of 63 hours; decreased to 24 to 63 hours with coadministration of other antiepileptics; peaks in 2 to 6 hours; reaches steady state in 14 days

Dispensing
Q.i.d. or b.i.d.; dose reduction or discontinuation should be done gradually

Range of Dosing
Adults: initiate therapy with 100 mg per day for 2 weeks. Increase dose by 100 mg per day every 2 weeks up to 400 mg per day. Effective range is 100 to 600 mg per day; no suggestion of increased response with doses greater than 400 mg per day.

Children: safety and efficacy for children younger than 16 years have not been established.

Elderly: more likely to have decreased renal function and creatinine clearance; consider renal function monitoring. Increased AUC by 35% with creatinine clearance less than 20 mL per minute.

FDA Approval
Adjuvant therapy in treatment of partial seizures in adults with epilepsy; **not approved** for pediatric patients younger than 16 years.

Possible Mechanism of Action
- Inhibits voltage-dependent sodium currents and T-type calcium channels to suppress repetitive firing of neurons
- Blocks glutamate receptors to decrease excitation
- Enhances GABA-mediated inhibition to reduce hyperpolarization

Possible Advantages
May be neuroprotective due to decreased lipid peroxidation in cortex and decreased glutamate excitotoxicity, such as ischemic cerebral damage; prevents dopaminergic neurodegeneration and facilitates serotonergic neurotransmission

Side Effects
- Allergy/hypersensitivity
- Hematologic: ecchymosis, rash, pruritus, leukopenia

- Neurologic: depression; psychosis; psychomotor slowing, including speech and language difficulties; confusion; fatigue; somnolence; headache; tremor; incoordination
- Kidney stones
- In pediatric patients: oligohydrosis, hyperthermia
- Teratogenic

Metabolism and Drug Interaction

Reduced to 2-sulfamoylacetyl phenol by CYP 3A4; drugs that either induce or inhibit CYP 3A4 may alter serum concentration; excreted primarily in urine as parent compound and as the glucuronide of a metabolite

Tests

Monitor renal function; alkaline phosphatase, BUN, and creatine clearance in renally impaired and elderly patients.

Anxiolytics/Sedative-Hypnotics

BENZODIAZEPINES

Chemical Group

BZDs, example: 8-chloro-1-methyl-6-phenyl-4H-s-triazolo[4,3-a]
[1,4]benzodiazepine(alprazolam)

Trade Names

Refer to Table 7.1 for trade names.

Pharmacokinetics

Due to different chemical structures, BZDs vary in their pharmacokinetic properties (Table 7.2).

Dispensing

Refer to Table 7.1 for dispensing information.

Range of Dosing

Refer to Table 7.1 for dose ranges.

Possible Mechanism of Action

- Bind to a specific site on $GABA_A$ receptors
- Linked to, but distinct from, the GABA receptor recognition site
- Enhances GABA recognition, potentiating inhibitory action

Possible Advantages

- Wide range of selection (Table 7.1) to benefit individual patient,
  minimizing adverse effects due to different pharmacokinetic
  properties
- Effective in several anxiety and sleep disorders, as well as in
  anxiety and agitation associated with other disorders
- Safe in overdose if used alone

Side Effects

- Sedation—initially, but often subsides as anxiolytic action sets
  in
- Behavioral disinhibition
- Psychomotor impairment—coordination and sustained atten-
  tion
- Cognitive impairment—even with a single dose
- Confusion, ataxia, excitement, agitation, transient hypoten-
  sion, vertigo, and GI distress in some patients
- Psychological habituation, physical dependence
- For all sedative-hypnotics: anaphylaxis, angioedema, and com-
  plex sleep-related behaviors

Withdrawal Symptoms

Although BZDs can produce dependence, hence withdrawal
symptoms, this is unlikely with short-term use. Withdrawal is
more likely when higher potency BZDs are taken for a longer
duration and discontinued abruptly.

Table 7.1. Commonly used benzodiazepines

	Generic Name	Trade Name	Half-life, Including Metabolite (hr)	Lipid Solubility	Active Metabolite	Dose Range
Intermediate to long acting	Diazepam[a]	Valium	20–70	High	Yes	5–100 mg/d
	Lorazepam[a]	Ativan	10–70	Moderate	No	1–6 mg/d
	Clonazepam[a]	Klonopin	19–50	Moderate	No	1–6 mg/d
Short to intermediate acting	Alprazolam[a]	Xanax	8–15	Moderate	No	0.5–6 mg/d
	Oxazepam[a]	Serax	5–15	Moderate	No	5–60 mg/d
	Temazepam[b]	Restoril	8–12	High	No	15–45 mg/d
	Midazolam[a]	Versed	1.5–3.5	High	No	5–15 mg/IV dose

[a]Most frequently used as anxiolytic.
[b]Most frequently used as hypnotic.

Table 7.2.   Pharmacokinetic properties of benzodiazepines

Properties	Short Acting	Long Acting
Potency	High	Low
Daily dosage frequency	Q4–6 hr	b.i.d. or once daily
Interdose anxiety	Frequent	Rare
Accumulation	Little or none	Common
Hypnotic hangover effects	None or mild	Mild to moderate
Rebound anxiety	Frequent	Infrequent
Dependency risk	High	Low
Onset withdrawal symptoms	1–3 d	4–7 d
Duration withdrawal symptoms	2–5 d	8–15 d
Paradoxical effects	Frequent	Infrequent
Anterograde amnesia	Frequent	Infrequent
IM administration	Rapid absorption	Slow absorption
IV risk	Low	High with rapid injection
Active metabolites	None or few	Many

Source: Adapted from Janicak PG, Davis JM, Perskorn SH, et al. *Principles and Practice of Psychopharmacotherapy.* 4th ed. Philadelphia: Lippincott Williams & Wilkins; 2006.

Symptoms
- Various GI symptoms
- Diaphoresis
- Tremor, lethargy, dizziness, headaches
- Increased acuity for smell and sound
- Restlessness, insomnia, irritability, anxiety
- Tinnitus
- Feelings of depersonalization
- Seizures, especially with abrupt withdrawal of high-potency BZD (e.g., alprazolam)

Tapering
It is important to taper the BZD dose to avoid withdrawal symptoms (necessary in patients who have taken a BZD for more than 4 months, especially with potent, short-acting BZD). History of seizures is another important reason to slowly taper BZD.

BUSPIRONE

Chemical Group
Azaspirodecanedione

Trade Name
Buspar (Bristol-Myers Squibb); generic buspirone (Mylan Pharmaceuticals, Teva, Actavis Towato, Ethex, Ivax, Ranbaxy, Datian)

Forms Available
Tablets of 5, 10, and 15 mg, 30 mg (scored)

Pharmacokinetics
Half-life 5 to 11 hours; bioavailability increased with food

Dispensing
T.i.d.

Range of Dosing
Adults: start with 5 mg t.i.d.; maximum effect in 4 to 6 weeks; can be discontinued abruptly.
Children: the very young can begin at 2.5 mg t.i.d. and increase to 5 mg t.i.d. (given at 0.2 to 1 mg per kg per day).
Elderly: start at 5 mg b.i.d.; may increase to maximum of 60 mg per day. Anxiolytic effect at low dose unpredictable; modest agitation effects at higher doses

FDA Approval
GAD

Possible Mechanism of Action:
- $5HT_{1a}$ receptor partial agonist: decreases 5HT turnover
- 1-Phenyl-piperazine metabolite—acts via α_2 adrenergic receptors, increase firing rate in locus coeruleus

Possible Advantages
No dependency problems, sedation, or psychomotor retardation; safe in overdose

Side Effects
- Headache, GI distress, dizziness
- Anaphylaxis, angioedema, and complex sleep-related behaviors
- Less useful in persons who have been on BZDs

Drug Interactions
- Avoid use with MAOIs
- Inhibitors of CYP 3A4, such as grapefruit juice, diltiazem, erythromycin, and itraconazole, may elevate levels of buspirone.

PREGABALIN

Chemical Group
S-3-(aminomethyl)-5-methylhexanoic acid

Trade Name
Lyrica (Pfizer)

Forms Available
Capsules of 25, 50, 75, 100, 150, 200, 225, and 300 mg

Pharmacokinetics
Half-life is ~6 hours; greater than 90% is eliminated unchanged in the urine; is not bound to plasma proteins; steady-state concentration (c_{ss}) achieved in 1 to 2 days after repeated dosing

Dispensing
B.i.d or t.i.d. When discontinuing, taper gradually over a minimum of 1 week.

Range of Dosing
- *Adults:* start at 50 mg t.i.d. (150 mg per day); increase to 400 to 600 mg per day based on efficacy and tolerance.
- *Children:* little information available
- *Elderly:* start at 50 mg t.i.d.; increased according to tolerance and efficacy. Because of age-related renal impairment, appropriate dosage adjustment is recommended.

FDA Approval
Neuropathic pain
As an adjunct for adults with partial onset seizures
GAD (anticipating approval)

Possible Mechanism of Action
- Presynaptic binding to the alpha-2-delta subunit of voltage-sensitive calcium channels reduces depolarization-induced calcium influx.
- May modulate release of sensory neuropeptide substance P and calcitonin gene-related peptide

Possible Advantages
- No dependence
- No hepatic drug–disease or drug–drug interactions

Side Effects
- Dizziness, drowsiness (greater than 10%)
- Visual disturbances, ataxia, dysarthria, euphoria, edema (1% to 10%)
- Anaphylaxis, angioedema, and complex sleep-related behaviors
  (See also discussion of SSRIs, venlafaxine, and duloxetine as treatments for anxiety disorders.)

ZOLPIDEM

Chemical Group
Imidazopyridine

Trade Name
Ambien (Searle); generic Zolpidem (Mylan, Teva, Roxane, and several others)

Forms Available
Tablets: 5 and 10 mg
XR tablets: 6.25 and 12.5 mg

Pharmacokinetics
Half-life is 2.4 hours in adults; rapidly absorbed after oral administration; high plasma protein binding capacity; peak blood levels reached in 2.2 hours; 6 to 8 hours of duration of action

Dispensing
Once daily QHS

Range of Dosing
Adults: 2.5 to 10 mg immediately before bedtime. Maximum dose recommended is 10 mg.
Children: no information available
Elderly: 2.5 to 5 mg immediately before bedtime, maximum dose should not exceed 10 mg. Insufficient data to conclude that cognitive function is not impaired in the elderly.

FDA Approval
Short-term treatment of insomnia

Possible Mechanism of Action
Non-BZD hypnotic that acts selectively on the alpha-subunit of the GABA-BZ receptor complex. Modulation of these chloride-receptor channels potentiates the inhibitory effect of GABA.

Possible Advantages
- No muscle relaxant, anxiolytic, or anticonvulsant effects with sedative dose
- Less likely to affect sleep architecture
- No or minimal rebound withdrawal effects
- Less abuse potential than with BZDs

Side Effects
1% to 10%

- CNS: headache, drowsiness, dizziness
- GI: nausea, diarrhea, vomiting
- Neuromuscular and skeletal: myalgia; less than 1%—amnesia, confusion, falls, tremor
- May cause memory impairment
- Anaphylaxis, angioedema, and complex sleep-related behaviors

Metabolism and Drug Interactions

- Metabolized in liver; therefore, dose adjustment required in hepatically impaired and elderly persons
- Increased effect or toxicity with alcohol, CNS depressants, and SSRIs
- Contraindicated during lactation

ZALEPLON

Chemical Group
Pyrazolopyrimidine derivative

Trade Name
Sonata (Wyeth-Ayerst); generic Zaleplon (Seypharma, Teva)

Form Available
Capsules: 5 and 10 mg

Pharmacokinetics
Half-life is 1 hour; rapid onset with peak effect and peak serum concentration reached within 1 hour; duration of action 6 to 8 hours; absorption is rapid and almost complete with 30% bioavailability; high-fat meal can prolong absorption

Dispensing
Once daily, immediately before bedtime or when patient cannot fall asleep

Range of Dosing
Adults: 10 mg QHS; usual dose range is 5 to 20 mg
Children: no information available
Elderly: 5 mg QHS

FDA Approval
Short-term treatment of insomnia

Possible Mechanism of Action
Non-BZD hypnotic that acts selectively at omega-1 receptors on the alpha-subunit of the GABA-BZ receptor complex; modulation of these chloride-receptor channels potentiates the inhibitory effect of GABA

Possible Advantages
- Decreases sleep latency with minimal effect on sleep stages
- Due to its very short half-life, it is useful in patients with difficulty falling asleep, staying asleep, and going back to sleep after waking up at night.
- At the recommended dosage, cognitive and psychomotor skills are apparently not significantly impaired.
- Possible absence of rebound insomnia and withdrawal symptoms on discontinuation

Side Effects
>10%
- CNS: headache

1% to 10%
- CVS: peripheral edema
- CNS: amnesia, anxiety, depersonalization, hallucinations, somnolence, vertigo, depression, impaired coordination, dizziness, tremor, complex sleep-related behaviors
- Skin: rash, photosensitivity, angioedema, anaphylaxis

- GIT: abdominal pain, anorexia, colitis, dyspepsia, nausea, constipation
- Neuromuscular: myalgia, weakness

Caution

When used in patients:

- With depression, particularly with suicidal risk
- With history of drug dependence
- Performing tasks requiring mental alertness, such as operating heavy machinery or driving

Metabolism and Drug Interactions

- Zaleplon is primarily metabolized by aldehyde/oxidase and to a lesser extent by CYP 3A4.
- All metabolites are pharmacologically inactive.
- Zaleplon potentiates CNS effects of alcohol, imipramine, and thioridazine.
- Alternative drug is chosen if patient is taking CYP 3A4 inducers, such as phenytoin, carbamazepine, and phenobarbital.
- Lower doses of zaleplon are used when coprescribed with cimetidine (because cimetidine inhibits both aldehyde oxidase and CYP 3A4).

ESZOPLICONE

Chemical Group
Pyrrolopyrazine derivative of the cyclopyrrolone class (S-isomer of zopiclone)

Trade Name
Lunesta (Sepracor)

Form Available
Tablets of 1-, 2-, and 3-mg strength

Pharmacokinetics
Rapidly absorbed; effects may be reduced when taken with or immediately after a high-fat/heavy meal. C_{max} in ~1 hour; elimination half-life is 6 hours. Weakly protein bound (~52% to 59%).

Dispensing
Once daily at bedtime; should be taken only immediately prior to going to bed or after going to bed and experiencing difficulty falling asleep, because of the rapid onset of action

Range of Dosing
Adults: recommended start dose is 2 mg. Dosing may be initiated or increased to 3 mg if clinically indicated
Children: no experience available
Elderly: recommended starting dose for elderly persons whose primary complaint is difficulty falling asleep is 1 mg. Dose may be increased to 2 mg if clinically indicated. For elderly patients whose primary complaint is difficulty staying asleep, the recommended dose is 2 mg.

FDA Approval
Insomnia

Possible Mechanism of Action
• Binding with GABA-receptor complexes located close to or allosterically coupled to BZD receptors

Possible Advantages
• Facilitates sleep onset and sleep maintenance
• Unique in that it may be used longer term

Side Effects
• CNS: headache (21%); somnolence (10%); dizziness (7%); nervousness (5%); depression (4%); anxiety, confusion, hallucinations, decreased libido, abnormal dreams, neuralgia (3%); migraine (at least 1%)
• Dermatologic: rash, pruritus (4%)
• GI: unpleasant taste (34%); dry mouth (7%); dyspepsia, nausea (5%); diarrhea (4%); vomiting (3%)
• Genitourinary: dysmenorrhea, gynecomastia, UTI (3%)
• Respiratory: respiratory infection (10%)

- Miscellaneous: pain (5%); accidental injury, viral infection (3%); chest pain, peripheral edema (at least 1%), anaphylaxis, angioedema, complex sleep-related behaviors

Contraindications
None known

Precautions
- Hepatic: start dose should be 1 mg in patients with severe hepatic impairment (should be used with caution in these patients).

Metabolism and Drug Interactions
- Metabolism is by CYP 3A4 and CYP 2E1 via demethylation and oxidation
- No inhibitory potential on CYP450, 1A2, 2A6, 2C9, 2C19, and 2D6
- Elimination by kidneys, primarily as metabolites
- CYP 3A4 and CYP 2E1 substrate inducers may decrease effect, and inhibitors may increase effect or adverse effects.

RAMELTEON

Chemical Group
Tricyclic indan derivative/TAK-375 (a tricyclic synthetic analog of melatonin)

Trade Name
Rozerem (Takeda)

Form Available
8 mg tablets

Pharmacokinetics
Rapidly absorbed; median peak concentration in 0.75 hours; 82% protein bound; elimination half-life is 1 to 2.5 hours

Dispensing
8 mg within 30 minutes of going to bed

Range of Dosing
Adults: 8 mg QHS
Children: no information available
Elderly: 8 mg QHS (usually recommended dose does not require modification in elderly)

FDA Approval
Insomnia characterized by sleep onset difficulty

Possible Mechanism of Action
Melatonin 1 and 2 receptor agonist

Anatomic Site of Action
Suprachiasmatic nucleus

Possible Advantages
- No dependence or potential for abuse;
- Currently, the only nonscheduled prescription drug approved for the treatment of insomnia;
- No withdrawal and rebound insomnia

Side Effects
- CNS: headache (7%); somnolence, dizziness (5%); fatigue (4%); exacerbated insomnia (3%); depression (2%)
- GI: nausea (3%); diarrhea, dysgeusia (2%)
- Laboratory tests: decreased blood cortisol (1%)
- Musculoskeletal: arthralgia, myalgia (2%)
- Respiratory: upper respiratory tract infection (3%); influenza (1%)

Contraindications
- Hypersensitivity to the drug or any of its components
- Severe hepatic impairment
- Patients taking fluvoxamine

Metabolism and Drug Interactions

- CYP 1A2 is the major isoenzyme involved in the metabolism.
- Should be administered with extreme caution in patients taking other CYP 1A2 inhibitors, strong CYP 2C9 inhibitors, and strong CYP 3A4 inhibitors.
- When used with potent CYP enzyme inducers, efficacy of ramelteon may be decreased due to decreases in the concentration.

Adjuvant Medications

CLONIDINE

Chemical Group
Imidazoline

Trade Name
Catapres (Boehringer-Ingelheim); generic clonidine (Apotex Incorporated, Novopharm Limited)

Forms Available
Patches: 0.1, 0.2, and 0.3 mg per day per week
Tablets: 0.1, 0.2, and 0.3 mg
Epidural injection in 10-mL vial of 1 mg

Pharmacokinetics
Half-life 9 hours; peaks in 1 to 3 hours

Dispensing
B.i.d. Tablet must be split first and must be used 0.05 mg b.i.d.

Range of Dosing
Adults: 0.1 mg b.i.d. to t.i.d. is safe. Always consider tapering the dose.
Children: start at 0.05 mg per day or b.i.d., depending on weight and severity of problem. Titrate during week 1 to a maximum of 0.1 mg t.i.d.
Elderly: start at low end of dose range; can be increased to adult levels. Clonidine has few metabolic and serious side effects and has a relatively low cost, which may make it a useful choice for the elderly. Hypotension is a possibility.

FDA Approval
Hypertension, treatment of severe pain in cancer patients (combined with opiates)

Possible Mechanism of Action
Centrally acting, alpha-agonist

Possible Advantages
- Opioid withdrawal: decreases autonomic hyperarousal
- Gilles de la Tourette's syndrome: 2 to 3 months to assess benefit; 0.1 to 0.3 mg per day
- Akathisia: 0.1 to 0.2 mg per day
- First used for tics, then for ADHD, PTSD, to induce sleep, and ANS hyperarousal
- Safe up to 0.1 mg t.i.d.

Side Effects
- Sedation
- Hypotension

- Rebound hypertension (tolerance may develop in 2 weeks)
- Dry mouth, eyes
- Nausea and vomiting
- Rash
- Impotence
- Postural dizziness
- Vivid dreams
- Insomnia
- Anxiety/depression
- Gynecomastia
- Children develop allergy to patches; cream can help

Metabolism and Drug Interactions

- Lipophilic, penetrates blood–brain barrier
- 50% excreted by kidneys, 50% by liver
- Tricyclics can decrease the effect of clonidine.

GUANFACINE

Chemical Group
Acetamide hydrochloride

Trade Name
Tenex (Robins)

Forms Available
Tablets: 1 and 2 mg

Pharmacokinetics
Half-life is 10 to 30 hours; younger patients have shorter half-life (13 to 14 hours); older patients have half-life at upper end of range.

Dispensing
Q.i.d.

Range of Dosing
Adults: recommended initial dose of 1 mg per day; maximum dose of 4 mg per day
Children: recommended maximum dose is 3 mg per day.
Elderly: dose adjustment is not required. Age reduction in urinary excretion and renal clearance was observed in the elderly and was accompanied by an increase in proportion of metabolites. Based on these studies and dual renal and nonrenal clearance, the dose usually does not need to be adjusted.

FDA Approval
Hypertension

Possible Mechanism of Action
Centrally acting antihypertensive with α_2 adrenoreceptor agonist action

Possible Advantages
- Opioid withdrawal: decreases autonomic hyperarousal
- Gilles de la Tourette's syndrome: 2 to 3 months to assess benefit; 0.1 to 0.3 mg per day
- Akathisia: 0.1 to 0.2 mg per day
- Given the longer half-life, midday dose can be avoided (unlike clonidine).

Side Effects
- Sedation
- Hypotension
- Dry mouth, eyes
- Nausea
- Impotence
- Postural dizziness
- Vivid dreams
- Insomnia
- Anxiety/depression

- Rebound hypertension (delayed compared with clonidine, consistent with its longer half-life)

Metabolism and Drug Interactions

- Guanfacine and its metabolites are excreted primarily in urine.
- ~50% of dose is eliminated unchanged in urine.
- Increased sedation occurs when given with other CNS–depressant drugs.

Psychostimulants

METHYLPHENIDATE

Chemical Group
Piperidine derivative

Trade Name
Ritalin (Novartis); generic methylphenidate (such as Methylin, etc.) (MallincKrodt Inc, Alliant Pharmaceuticals)

Forms Available
Tablets: 5, 10, and 20 mg, and 20 mg SR (SR; only as Ritalin, not generic)

Pharmacokinetics
Half-life is 2 to 3 hours; peaks in 1.5 to 2.5 hours; entirely excreted in urine in 12 to 24 hours. Behavioral effects occur within 30 to 60 minutes; peak in 1 to 3 hours; dissipates in 3 to 5 hours. SR effects are seen in 1 to 2 hours; peak in 3 to 5 hours; lasts for 8 hours.

Dispensing
Usually 8 AM, 12 PM, and 4 PM, if required.

Range of Dosing
Children: Lower doses (0.3 mg per kg) were believed to be most helpful for learning, whereas higher doses were found to be better for social behavior. Maximum dosing is 1 mg per kg. There are significant differences in response across individuals. A safe maximum dose is 40 to 60 mg per day.
Adults: 0.5 mg per kg body weight
Elderly: no information available

FDA Approval
ADHD, narcolepsy

Possible Mechanism of Action
Enhances release of DA and, to a lesser extent, NE

Possible Advantages
• Improves vigilance, impulse control, fine motor coordination, and reaction time
• Reduces task-irrelevant responses and improves persistence
• Reduces aggression, impulsive behavior, noisiness, noncompliance, and disruptiveness
• Improves quality of social interactions with peers, parents, and teachers

Side Effects
• Decreased appetite, sleeplessness, anxiety/irritability/crying (mood symptoms may be associated with the disorder); may

be more evident in the washout time rather than in the peak plasma level period
- Stomach aches/headaches may be reported, but tend to be mild.
- Tics in 1%, exacerbated in 13%
- Behavioral rebound
- Drug dependence, height and weight suppression
- Sudden death with pre-existing structural cardiac abnormalities

Metabolism and Drug Interactions
- Mainly metabolized to ritalinic acid and is pharmacologically inactive
- Cumulative effect with other stimulant medications and MAOIs

Tests
Baseline ECG

CONCERTA, EXTENDED RELEASE

Chemical Group
Methylphenidate hydrochloride, piperidine derivative

Trade Name
Concerta (ALZA Pharmaceuticals)

Forms Available
Tablets: 18, 26, 36, and 54 mg

Pharmacokinetics
Half-life is 12 hours. Initial peak level is reached in 1 to 2 hours and gradually increases over the next few hours. Peak plasma level is reached in 6 to 8 hours. Concerta uses osmotic pressure to deliver methylphenidate at a controlled rate. The tablet has an osmotically active trilayer core surrounded by a semipermeable membrane with an IR drug overcoat. There is a laser-drilled orifice on the push layer (outer layer of the trilayer core) at the drug layer end of the tablet. As water enters the tablet in the stomach, methylphenidate is released from the tablet through the orifice. The membrane controls the osmotic rate and drug delivery.

Dispensing
Single AM dose. No evidence of dose dumping with food.
- 15 mg per day of regular tablets of methylphenidate, or 20 mg SR
- 30 mg per day of regular tablets of methylphenidate, or 40 mg SR
- 45 mg per day of regular tablets of methylphenidate, or 60 mg SR

Range of Dosing
Children: lower doses (0.3 mg per kg) were believed to help the most for learning, whereas higher doses were found to be better for social behavior. Maximum dosing is 1 mg per kg per day. There are significant differences in response across individuals. It has not been studied for children younger than 6 years of age.
Adults: 0.5 mg per kg body weight
Elderly: no information available

FDA Approval
ADHD

Possible Mechanism of Action
Enhances NE and DA release; more effect on DA than d-amphetamine

Possible Advantages
Single dose resulting in smooth effect throughout the day; there is no need to take it at school or work

Side Effects

Headache, abdominal pain, nausea, loss of appetite, tremors, tics, high blood pressure, insomnia

Contraindications

Tics, anxiety/agitation, glaucoma

Metabolism and Drug Interactions

- Mainly metabolized to ritalinic acid, which is pharmacologically inactive
- Additive effects with other stimulant medications and MAOIs

Tests

Baseline ECG, CBC, complete metabolic profile (CMP)

METHYLPHENIDATE TRANSDERMAL SYSTEM

Chemical Group
Piperidine derivative

Trade Name
Daytrana (Shire Pharmaceuticals)

Forms Available
Patches consisting of 27.5 mg, 41.3 mg, 55.0 mg, and 82.5 mg

Pharmacokinetics
Half-life in children aged 6 to 12 years was approximately 3 to 4 hours (mean peak concentration of 39 ng/mL in 7.5 to 10.5 hours).

Dispensing
A patch, which consists of three layers—an outside backing; an adhesive containing methylphenidate; and a protective liner—is applied to hip (alternating) for 9 hours, usually in the AM.

Range of Dosing
Children: 10 mg per 9 hours, 15 mg per 9 hours, 20 mg per 9 hours, and 30 mg per 9 hours (not studied in children under 6 years of age)
Adults: No information is available.
Elderly: No information is available.

FDA Approval
ADHD (in children)

Possible Mechanism of Action
Blocks the reuptake of NE and DA into the presynaptic neuron and increases the release of these monoamines into the extraneuronal space

Possible Advantages
- Improves vigilance, impulse control, fine motor coordination, and reaction time
- Reduces task-irrelevant responses and improves persistence
- Reduces aggression, impulsive behavior, noisiness, noncompliance, and disruptiveness
- Improves quality of social interactions with peers, parents, and teachers

Side Effects
- Contact sensitization
- Headaches
- Depression, fatigue
- Hypertension and other cardiovascular disorders

Contraindications
Agitation, hypersensitivity to methylphenidate, glaucoma, tics, MAOIs

Metabolism

Methylphenidate is metabolized primarily by de-esterification to alpha-phenyl-piperidine acetic acid (ritalinic acid), which has little or no pharmacologic activity. Transdermal administration of methylphenidate exhibits much less first-pass effect than does oral administration.

Drug Interactions

MAOIs, hypertensive medications, coumarin anticoagulants, anticonvulsants (e.g., phenobarbital, phenytoin, primidone), some tricyclic drugs (e.g., imipramine, clomipramine, desipramine), SSRIs, and clonidine

Tests

Baseline ECG, CBC, CMP

METADATE CONTROLLED DELIVERY

Chemical Group
Methylphenidate HCL, piperidine derivative

Trade Name
Metadate CD (Celltech Pharmaceuticals, Inc.)

Form Available
Capsules of 10, 20, 30, 40, 50, and 60 mg

Pharmacokinetics
Methylphenidate HCL, ER capsules. Diffucaps technology was used. The capsules contain two kinds of beads: the IR and ER beads. Thirty percent of the dose (6 mg) is provided by the IR beads and 70% of the dose (14 mg) by the ER beads. The continued release beads each have an additional ethyl cellulose coating that provides ER characteristics. The first peak plasma level is reached in 1.5 hours; the second peak is reached in 4.5 hours. The beads contain an aqueous outer protective membrane in addition to the release control membrane in ER beads. Half-life is 6.8 hours.

Dispensing
Single AM dose before breakfast

Range of Dosing
Children: start at 20 mg. Raise dose only in 20-mg increments; never more than 60 mg. Conversion is equivalent to standard form of methylphenidate.
Adults: 0.5 to 1 mg per kg body weight
Elderly: no information available

FDA Approval
ADHD

Possible Mechanism of Action
Enhances release of DA and, to a lesser extent, NE

Possible Advantages
• Single ER dosing
• Long-term effects and efficacy not yet tested

Side Effects
• Decreased appetite, sleeplessness, anxiety/irritability/crying (mood symptoms may be associated with the disorder)
• Stomach aches/headaches may be reported, but tend to be mild.
• Elevated blood pressure
• Behavioral rebound
• Drug dependence, height and weight suppression
• Seizures (particularly in patients with prior EEG abnormalities)
• Sudden death has been reported in association with CNS stimulant treatment at usual doses in children and adolescents with structural cardiac abnormalities.

Contraindications
Tics, anxiety/agitation, glaucoma

Metabolism and Drug Interactions
- Mainly metabolized to ritalinic acid, which is pharmacologically inactive
- Additive effects with other stimulant medications and MAOIs
- Fruit juices and ascorbic acid decrease absorption.

Tests
Baseline ECG, CBC, CMP

DEXMETHYLPHENIDATE

Chemical Group
This is the d- or "right-handed" isomer of the racemic mixture found in d,1-methylphenidate. The active isomer is isolated as dexmethylphenidate.

Trade Name
Focalin (Novartis)
Focalin XR (Novartis)

Forms Available
Tablets: 2.5, 5, 7.5, and 10 mg; tablets XR: 5 mg, 10 mg, 15 mg, and 20 mg

Pharmacokinetics
Half-life is 2 to 5 hours; reaches peak in 1 to 4 hours; entirely excreted in urine within 12 to 24 hours. Behavioral effects occur within 30 to 60 minutes; peak in 1 to 4 hours; dissipate in 3 to 5 hours. Focalin XR produces a bimodal plasma concentration-time profile (i.e., two distinct peaks approximately 4 hours apart). The first peak concentration is reached in 1.5 hours (typical range 1 to 4 hours). The time to the second peak is slightly longer for Focalin XR given once daily (about 6.5 hours, range 4.5 to 7 hours) compared to Focalin tablets given in two doses 4 hours apart.

Dispensing
Focalin tablet is given as b.i.d., at least 4 hours apart. Focalin XR is an ER formulation with a bimodal release profile that uses SODAS (Spheroidal Oral Drug Absorption System) technology. Each capsule contains the half dose as IR and the other half as a second delayed release of the drug. XR is given as a single dose.

Range of Dosing
Children: starting dose is 2.5 mg. Maximum recommended dose is 20 mg per day. Patients being switched from methylphenidate should be started at half their final methylphenidate dose because it is more active.
Adults: 0.5 mg per kg per day
Elderly: no information available

FDA Approval
ADHD

Possible Mechanism of Action
Enhances DA and, to a lesser extent, NE release

Possible Advantages
* Improves vigilance, impulse control, fine motor coordination, and reaction time
* Reduces task-irrelevant responses and improves persistence
* Reduces aggression, impulsive behavior, noisiness, noncompliance, and disruptiveness
* Improves quality of social interactions with peers, parents, and teachers

- Efficacy is considered superior to that of methylphenidate because it is the active isomer.

Side Effects

- Decreased appetite, sleeplessness, anxiety/irritability/crying (mood symptoms may be associated with the disorder); may be more problematic in the washout than in the peak period
- Stomach aches/headaches may be reported, but tend to be mild.
- Tics in 1%, exacerbated in 13%
- Behavioral withdrawal rebound
- Concerns about drug dependence, height and weight suppression, and heart problems are not supported by existing data.

Metabolism and Drug Interactions

- Mainly metabolized to ritalinic acid, which is pharmacologically inactive
- Additive effect with other stimulant medications and MAOIs

Tests

Baseline ECG, periodic CBC, differential, and platelet counts

DEXTROAMPHETAMINE

Chemical Group
Dextroamphetamine sulfate

Trade Name
Dexedrine (tablets and spansules) (Smith-Kline-Beecham) and DextroStat (tablets) (Shire Richwood, Inc.)

Forms Available
Dexedrine: tablets 5, 10, and 15 mg; Dexedrine spansule: capsules of 5, 10, and 15 mg; elixir 5 mg per 5 mL; DextroStat: tablets of 5 and 10 mg

Pharmacokinetics
Half-life is 4 to 6 hours; reaches peak in 1.5 to 2.5 hours. Behavioral effects occur within 30 to 60 minutes; peak in 1 to 3 hours; dissipated in 4 to 6 hours. Dexedrine spansule peaks in 8 to 10 hours.

Dispensing
Usually 8 AM, 12 PM, and 4 PM (if required)

Range of Dosing
Children: lower doses (0.15 mg per kg) were believed to be better for learning, whereas higher doses were found to be better for social behavior. Maximum dosing is 1.5 mg per kg per day. Safe maximum dose is 30 mg per day. There are significant differences in response across individuals.
Adults: 0.25 to 0.5 mg per kg body weight.
Elderly: No dose recommendations are available. Some physicians see benefits as an antidepressant for elderly patients who cannot tolerate the side effects of traditional therapy. Benefits are usually noted within 36 hours, and habituation is generally not a problem.

FDA Approval
ADHD, narcolepsy

Possible Mechanism of Action
Sympathomimetic that enhances NE and DA release

Possible Advantages
- Improves vigilance, impulse control, fine motor coordination, and reaction time
- Reduces task-irrelevant responses and improves persistence
- Reduces aggression, impulsive behavior, noisiness, noncompliance, and disruptiveness
- Improves quality of social interactions with peers, parents, and teachers

Side Effects

- Decreased appetite, sleeplessness, anxiety/irritability/crying (mood symptoms may be associated with the disorder); may be more problematic in the washout than in the peak period
- Stomach aches/headaches may be reported, but tend to be mild.
- Tics in 1%, exacerbated in 13%
- Behavioral rebound
- Drug dependence and cardiovascular problems have been reported in children and adolescents with pre-existing conditions.

Metabolism and Drug Interactions

- Mainly metabolized to benzoic acid in liver; excreted in urine within 24 hours
- Additive effect with other stimulant medications and MAOIs

Tests

Baseline ECG

ADDERALL

Chemical Group
Stimulant: dextroamphetamine sulfate and amphetamine sulfate with the dextro isomer of amphetamine saccharate and d,1-amphetamine aspartate

Trade Name
Adderall, Adderall XR (Shire Richwood, Inc.)

Forms Available
Tablets: 5, 7.5, 10, 12.5, 15, 20, and 30 mg; XR in capsules: 5, 10, 15, 20, 25, and 30 mg

Pharmacokinetics
Half-life is 2 to 3 hours; peaks in 1.5 to 2.5 hours; entirely excreted in urine by 12 to 24 hours. Behavioral effects occur within 30 to 60 minutes; peak in 1 to 3 hours; dissipate in 3 to 5 hours; peaks in 3 to 5 hours; lasts for 8 hours. Adderall XR peaks in 3 hours and takes 7 hours to reach maximum plasma concentration. Adderall XR contains two kinds of beads designed to give a double-pulsed delivery of amphetamine. Opening the capsule and sprinkling the contents on applesauce results in comparable absorption to the intact capsule taken in the fasted state. Sprinkle form must be consumed immediately and must not be chewed. Food prolongs the time to peak concentration (T_{max}) by 2.5 hours.

Dispensing
Usually 8 AM and 3 PM (if required)

Range of Dosing
Children: older than 3 years, range is between 2.5 and 30 mg per day, depending on age, weight, and response; weight-calculated dose is 0.15 to 0.2 mg per kg, or a maximum of 40 mg per day; Adderall XR recommended maximum dose is 30 mg per day
Adults: 0.25 to 0.5 mg per kg per day
Elderly: no information available

FDA Approval
ADHD, narcolepsy

Possible Mechanism of Action
Enhances NE and DA release

Possible Advantages
- Improves vigilance, impulse control, fine motor coordination, and reaction time
- Reduces task-irrelevant responses and improves persistence
- Reduces aggression, impulsive behavior, noisiness, noncompliance, and disruptiveness
- Improves quality of social interactions with peers, parents, and teachers
- May be superior in efficacy to other amphetamines

Side Effects

- Tachycardia and elevation of blood pressure
- Decreased appetite, sleeplessness, anxiety/irritability/crying (mood symptoms may be associated with the disorder)
- Stomachaches/headaches are reported, but tend to be mild.
- Tics in 1%, exacerbated in 13%
- Behavioral rebound
- Drug dependence
- Height and weight suppression and cardiovascular problems are associated in patients with pre-existing conditions.

Metabolism and Drug Interactions

- Mainly metabolized to ritalinic acid, which is pharmacologically inactive
- Additive effect with other stimulant medications and MAOIs
- Fruit juices and ascorbic acid decrease absorption.

Tests

Baseline ECG

MODAFINIL

Chemical Group

2-[(diphenylmethyl)sulfinyl]acetamide

Trade Name

Provigil (Cephalon)

Forms Available

Capsules of 100- and 200-mg strength

Pharmacokinetics

Absorption is rapid, with C_{max} occurring at 2 to 4 hours. Food slows absorption, but does not affect the total AUC. It is well distributed with an apparent volume of distribution ($\sim$0.9 L per kg) larger than the volume of total body water (0.6 L per kg). Half-life is 10 to 12 hours. Steady states are reached after 2 to 4 days. Modafinil is a racemic compound the enantiomers of which have different pharmacokinetics. Trough concentrations of the circulating drug after dosing consist of 90% of the L-isomer and 10% of the D-isomer.

Dispensing

Once-a-day dosing

Range of Dosing

Adults: Recommended dose is 200 mg once a day. For patients with narcolepsy and obstructive sleep apnea/hypopnea syndrome (OSAHS), the drug should be taken as a single dose in the morning. For patients with shift work sleep disorder (SWSD), the drug should be taken 1 hour prior to the start of their work shift.

Children: Safety and efficacy in individuals younger than 16 years have not been established.

Elderly: Safety and effectiveness in individuals older than 65 years have not been established. Increased incidence of adverse effects is shown to occur.

FDA Approval

Narcolepsy, SWSD, OSAHS; as an adjunctive to standard treatment(s)

Possible Mechanism of Action

Precise mechanism is unknown. Proposed to act by a synergistic combination of mechanisms including direct inhibition of DA and NE reuptake, as well as orexin (also known as hypocretins) activation

Possible Advantages

Not addictive; less abuse potential

Side Effects

- More common: headache, nausea, anxiety, nervousness, depression, diarrhea, difficulty sleeping, dizziness, dry mouth,

infection, loss of appetite, loss of muscle strength, prickling or tingling feeling, runny nose, sore throat
- Less common: abnormal ejaculation, amnesia, asthma, chest pain, chills, confusion, difficulty breathing, difficulty urinating, face muscle spasms, fainting, fever, gum inflammation, herpes simplex, high blood pressure, irregular heartbeat, joint difficulties, low blood pressure, loss of muscle coordination, mood swings, mouth ulcer, neck pain, nosebleed, stiff neck, tense muscles, thirst, tremor, vision problems, vomiting

Contraindications
- Hypersensitivity to the drug or other constituents of the tablet
- Previous cardiovascular problems, particularly while using other stimulants
- Cardiac conditions, particularly:
  - Left ventricular hypertrophy
  - Mitral valve prolapse

Pregnancy
Category C drug; should be used only if the potential benefit justifies the potential risk to the fetus. Caution should be exercised when administered to a nursing woman.

Precautions
- In patients engaged in potentially hazardous occupations (e.g., operating machinery or driving motor vehicles)
- In patients with severe hepatic insufficiency, with or without cirrhosis, the drug should be administered at a reduced dose.

Metabolism and Drug Interactions
- The major route of elimination (∼90%) is metabolism, primarily by the liver, with subsequent renal elimination of the metabolites. Metabolism occurs through hydrolytic deamidation, S-oxidation, aromatic ring hydroxylation, and glucuronide conjugation.
- Modafinil induces the cytochrome P450 enzymes CYP1A2, CYP2B6, and CYP3A4, as well as inhibiting CYP2C9 and CYP2C19.
- Potential interactions with drugs that inhibit, induce, or are metabolized by the cytochrome P450 isoenzymes and other hepatic enzymes.

ATOMOXETINE

Chemical Group
Benzenepropanamine, N-methyl-gamma-(2-methylphenoxy)-, hydrochloride

Trade Name
Strattera (Eli Lilly); generic Attentin (Torrent)

Forms Available
Capsule: 10, 18, 25, 40, 60, 80, and 100 mg
Generic Attentin: capsules of 10, 18, 25, 40, and 60 mg

Pharmacokinetics
Half-life is 5 hours. Peak level is reached in 1 to 2 hours after dosing. It is well absorbed after oral administration. Ninety-eight percent is primarily bound to albumin in plasma. Pharmacokinetic values were similar in adults and children older than 6 years when doses were normalized to a mg per kg basis.

Dispensing
Once daily or divided dose in morning and late afternoon or early evening) with food or without food; nausea/GI complaints may be reduced when given with food.

Range of Dosing
Adults: start at 40 mg per day. Dose can be increased after a minimum of 3 days and after 2 to 4 weeks if no optimal response is seen. Usual range is 60 to 120 mg per day with a mean dose of 95 mg per day, given in divided doses.
Children and adolescents (up to 70 kg body weight): start with 0.5 mg per kg per day. Dose can be increased after a minimum of 3 days 1.2 to 1.4 mg per kg per day or 100 mg, whichever is less.
Children and adolescents (more than 70 kg body weight): same as adults
Elderly: no information available

FDA Approval
ADHD in adults and children older than 6 years

Possible Mechanism of Action
Selective inhibition of presynaptic NE transporter

Possible Advantages
It is equipotent to methylphenidate. Further advantages need to be established.

Side Effects
- Dyspepsia, decreased appetite
- Headache, nausea, vomiting
- Fatigue, dizziness, insomnia, mood swings
- Impaired sexual function in adults with erectile disturbance and impotence
- Suicidal ideation in children and adolescents

Metabolism and Drug Interactions

Metabolized by CYP 2D6; drugs that inhibit CYP 2D6 such as fluoxetine, paroxetine, and quinidine can increase atomoxetine level.

Caution

Must be used cautiously with pressor agents, given the possibility of increased blood pressure. The capsule should not be broken and sprinkled on food (may cause irritation of mucosa and skin).

Contraindications

Atomoxetine should not be administered with or within 2 weeks of MAOI administration. Atomoxetine use with IV albuterol is contraindicated.

LISDEXAMFETAMINE DIMESYLATE

Chemical Group

Prodrug of dextroamphetamine (2S)-2, 6-diamino-N-[(1S)-1-methyl-2-phenylethyl] hexanamide dimethanesulfonate/L-lysine-d-amphetamine

Trade Name

Vyvanse (Shire/New River)

Forms Available

Capsules of 30, 50, and 70 mg

Pharmacokinetics

Rapidly absorbed from GIT after oral administration; can be taken with or without food. T_{max} is approximately 1 hour. Follows linear pharmacokinetics over the dose ranges of 30 to 70 mg.

Dispensing

Once a day oral administration (should be taken in the morning). Afternoon doses should be avoided because of the potential for insomnia.

Range of Dosing

Adults: 30 mg once a day in the morning; if needed, the dose may be increased once a week by 20 mg per day until symptoms improve or a maximum dose of 70 mg is reached.

Children: Recommended start dose is 30 mg once daily in the morning. If needed, the dose may be increased once a week until symptoms improve or a maximum dose of 70 mg is reached. Not recommended for children younger than 3 years. No studies in children under 6 years of age.

Elderly: Little information available

FDA Approval

ADHD

Possible Mechanism of Action

Converted to the active metabolite, dextroamphetamine, which blocks reuptake of NE and DA into the presynaptic neuron and increases release of the monoamines into extraneuronal space

Possible Advantages

• Less abuse potential
• Once-a-day dispensing

Side Effects

• CV: palpitations, tachycardia, elevation of blood pressure, myocardial infarction, sudden death
• Stomach pain
• Nausea and vomiting
• Dry mouth
• Dizziness
• Weight loss

- Trouble sleeping
- Irritability
- Decreased appetite

Contraindications

- Advanced atherosclerosis
- Symptomatic cardiovascular disease
- Moderate or severe hypertension
- Glaucoma
- Hyperthyroidism
- Agitated states
- History of drug abuse
- During or within 14 days following the administration of MAOI (hypertensive crisis may result)
- Known hypersensitivity or idiosyncrasy to sympathomimetic amines

Special Precautions

- Family history of sudden death or ventricular fibrillation
- Pre-existing hypertension (mild), heart failure, recent myocardial infarction (any condition that might be compromised by increases in heart rate or blood pressure)
- Pre-existing psychosis
- Tic disorders
- Seizure disorder
- Visual disturbances
- Engagement in potentially hazardous activities such as operating machinery or vehicles

Metabolism

Metabolized to dextroamphetamine and L-lysine by first-pass intestinal and/or hepatic metabolism; not metabolized by cytochrome P450 enzymes; inhibits monoamine oxidase; excreted primarily by kidneys. Elimination half-life averages less than 1 hour.

Drug Interactions

- Alpha blockers: inhibited by lisdexamfetamines.
- Antidepressants, tricyclics: lisdexamfetamines may enhance the activity of tricyclic antidepressants or sympathomimetic agents; d-dexamphetamine with desipramine or protriptyline and possibly other tricyclics cause striking and sustained increases in the concentration of d-amphetamine in the brain; cardiovascular side effects are potentiated.
- MAOIs: slow the metabolism of amphetamines, potentiating their action. This may result in hypertensive crisis. A variety of toxic neurologic effects and malignant hyperpyrexia can occur, sometimes with fatal results.
- Antihistamines: sedative effects of antihistaminics may be counteracted.
- Antihypertensives: hypotensive effects of antihypertensives may be antagonized by lisdexamfetamine.
- Chlorpromazine: blocks DA and NE receptors, thus inhibiting the central stimulant effects of amphetamines, and can be used to treat lisdexamfetamine poisoning.

Table 9.1. Most commonly used psychostimulants

Brand Name	Generic	Form	Dosage (mg)	Delivery System
Adderall XR	Mixed salts—dextro-amphetamine and amphetamine	Capsule	5, 10, 15, 20, 25, 30	Once daily or b.i.d. dosing. Bead delivery system with double-pulsed delivery. Peak is 3 hr, but maximum plasma concentration is 7 hr.
Dexedrine	Dextroamphetamine	Tablet, spanule, elixir	5, 10, 15 mg; 5 mg per mL	b.i.d. or t.i.d. Effect seen with in 30–60 min. Peak 1–3 hr with tablets Peak 8–10 hr for spanules
Vyvanse	Lisdexamfetamine dimesylate	Capsule (extended release)	30, 50, 70	Once daily
Ritalin*	Methylphenidate HCL	Tablet	5, 10, 20	Peaks in 1 hr Immediate release b.i.d. or t.i.d. Peaks in 1.9 hr
Ritalin SR†	Methylphenidate HCL	Tablet (sustained release)	20	Once per day or b.i.d. Effect lasts 8–12 hr Peaks in 4.7 hr
Ritalin LA	Methylphenidate HCL	Capsule (extended release)	20, 30, 40	Bimodal release profile, once-per-day dosing.
Methylin	Methylphenidate HCL	Tablet	5, 10, 20	Immediate release b.i.d. or t.i.d. Peaks in 1.9 hr
Methylin ER	Methylphenidate HCL	Tablet (extended release)	10, 20	b.i.d. or t.i.d. Effect lasts 8 hr Peaks in 4.7 hr

(continued)

Table 9.1. Most commonly used psychostimulants (*Continued*)

Brand Name	Generic	Form	Dosage (mg)	Delivery System
Metadate ER	Methylphenidate HCL	Tablet (extended release)	10, 20	b.i.d. or t.i.d. Effect lasts 8 hr
Metadate CD	Methylphenidate HCL	Diffucaps, bead delivery system	20	Bead delivery system Once per day or b.i.d. Effect lasts 8–12 hr Peaks in 2–4 hr
Concerta	Methylphenidate HCL	Tablet (extended release)	18, 36, 54	Osmotic pressure Once per day or b.i.d. Effect lasts 12 hr Peaks in 6 hr
Cylert	Methylphenidate HCL	Tablet	18.75, 37.5, 75	Once per day AM dose Peaks in 2–4 hr
Provigil	Modafinil	Tablet	100, 200	Once-per-day AM dose Peaks in 2–4 hr
Focalin	D-isomer of methylphenidate	Tablet	2.5, 5, 10	b.i.d. Peaks in 1–4 hr
Focalin XR	D-isomer of methylphenidate	Tablet (extended release)		Once per day (extended release) Peak is bimodal; once at 1.5 hr and again at 6.5 hr
Daytrana	Methylphenidate	Patch	27.5, 41.3, 55.0, 82.5 mg	Peaks in 7.5–10 hr; applied every 9 hr to alternating hips
Strattera	Atomoxetine HCL	Capsule	10, 18, 25, 40, 60, 80, 100	Once daily or divide dose in morning Peaks in 1–2 hr

*Ritalin 5 mg ~ Concerta 18 mg.
†Ritalin SR 20 mg ~ Concerta 18 mg; Ritalin SR, Metadate ER (bioequivalent).

- Lithium: inhibits the anorectic and stimulatory effects of the drug.
- Ethosuximide: intestinal absorption of ethosuximide may be delayed.
- Haloperidol: blocks DA receptors, thus inhibiting the central stimulant effects of amphetamines.
- Meperidine: D-amphetamines potentiate the analgesic effects of meperidine.
- Methenamine therapy: urinary excretion of amphetamines is increased, and efficacy is reduced, by acidifying agents used in methenamine therapy.
- NE: adrenergic effects are enhanced.
- Phenobarbital: intestinal absorption of phenobarbital may be delayed; coadministration may produce a synergistic anticonvulsant action.
- Phenytoin: intestinal absorption of phenytoin may be delayed; coadministration may produce a synergistic anticonvulsant action.
- Propoxyphene: in cases of overdose, amphetamine CNS stimulation is potentiated, and fatal convulsions can occur.

Drug/Laboratory Tests Interactions
- Interactions can cause significant elevation in plasma corticosteroid levels. The greatest increase is seen in the evening.
- Interference with urinary steroid determination may be encountered.

Tests
Before starting the drug
- Careful evaluation of history (including family history of sudden deaths or ventricular fibrillations, any other pre-existing psychiatric disorders)
- Thorough physical examination to assess for the presence of cardiac disease

After starting the drug
- Regular checks of blood, heart, and blood pressure
- Weight and height checkup in growing children

See Table 9.1 for most commonly used psychostimulants.

Drug Therapy for Substance Use Disorders

NALTREXONE

Chemical Group
Synthetic congener of oxymorphone (phenanthrene-containing opioid)

Trade Name
Nalorex, Revia (DuPont)

Forms Available
Tablets: 50 mg

Pharmacokinetics
Half-life of 4 hours; peak plasma level in 1 hour. Fifty mg of naltrexone can block the pharmacologic effects of 25 mg of IV) heroin for 24 hours. One hundred mg and 150 mg of naltrexone are effective for 48 and 72 hours, respectively.

Dispensing
QD

Range of Dosing
Alcoholism: 50 mg daily
Opioid dependence: Verify that patient has not used opioids in the last 7 to 10 days prior to initiating therapy. Confirmation is through urinalysis for opioids and/or a naloxone challenge test. Start therapy with an initial dose of 25 mg. If no signs of opiate withdrawal, then 50 mg per day thereafter. Alternative dosing schedules:

- 50 mg every weekday with 100 mg every Saturday
- 100 mg every other day
- 150 mg every third day

FDA Approval
Alcoholism (suppress cravings); opioid addiction (blocks effects of exogenously administered opioids)

Possible Mechanism of Action
Competitive blockade at CNS opiate receptors

Possible Advantages
- No development of tolerance or dependence
- Blocks physical dependence to heroin or morphine when coadministered with these agents

Side Effects
- Dose-related hepatotoxicity

- In alcoholism: nausea, headache, dizziness, anxiety, fatigue, insomnia, vomiting
- In opioid addiction: joint pain, muscle pain, abdominal pain/cramps, nausea, anxiety, vomiting, fatigue, rash, sexual dysfunction
- Opioid withdrawal symptoms may occur.

Metabolism and Drug Interactions

Extensive hepatic first-pass metabolism (bioavailability ranging from 5% to 40%) to form 6-beta-naltrexol; primarily excreted in urine

- More severe liver damage occurs when used with other hepatotoxic agents, such as disulfiram.
- Interaction with thioridazine causes increased somnolence and fatigue.
- Decreased effectiveness of opioid-containing medications (e.g., cough syrups, antidiarrheals, opioid analgesics).

Contraindications/Cautions

- Patients receiving opioid analgesics or currently taking opioids
- Patients in acute opioid withdrawal
- Acute hepatitis or liver failure
- Nursing mothers
- Safety and efficacy are yet to be established in patients younger than 18 years.

Tests

LFTs

NALTREXONE EXTENDED RELEASE

Chemical Group

Synthetic congener of oxymorphone (phenanthrene-containing opioid)

Trade Name

Vivitrol (Alkermes)

Pharmacokinetics

Vivitrol is an ER, microsphere formulation of naltrexone. After IM injection, the naltrexone plasma concentration time profile is characterized by a transient initial peak, which occurs approximately 2 hours after injection, followed by a second peak observed approximately 2 to 3 days later. Beginning approximately 14 days after dosing, concentrations slowly decline, with measurable levels for longer than 1 month. Elimination of naltrexone and its metabolites occurs primarily via urine, with minimal excretion of unchanged naltrexone. The elimination half-life of naltrexone following Vivitrol administration is 5 to 10 days.

Dispensing

Administered by an IM gluteal injection of a dosage strength of 380 mg per vial

Range of Dosing

IM injection every 4 weeks or once a month

FDA Approval

Alcohol dependence

Possible Mechanism of Action

Naltrexone is an opioid antagonist with highest affinity for the mu opioid receptor.

Possible Advantages

- Decrease in first-pass effect
- No development of tolerance or dependence
- Blocks physical dependence on heroin or morphine when coadministered with these agents

Side Effects

- Dose-related hepatotoxicity (potentially less than with oral formulation)
- In alcoholism: nausea, headache, dizziness, anxiety, fatigue, insomnia, vomiting
- In opioid addiction: joint pain, muscle pain, abdominal pain/cramps, nausea, anxiety, vomiting, fatigue, rash, sexual dysfunction
- Opioid withdrawal symptoms may occur
- Injection site reactions

Contraindications

- Patients receiving opioid analgesics or currently taking opioids
- Patients in acute opioid withdrawal

- Acute hepatitis or liver failure
- Nursing mothers
- Safety and efficacy are yet to be established in patients younger than 18 years.
- Any individual who has failed the naloxone challenge test or has a positive urine screen for opioids
- Patients who have previously exhibited hypersensitivity to naltrexone, PLG, carboxymethylcellulose, or any other components of the diluent

Metabolism

Hepatic metabolism to form 6-beta-naltrexol; primarily excreted in urine

- More severe liver damage when used with other hepatotoxic agents, such as disulfiram
- Interaction with thioridazine causes increased somnolence and fatigue.
- Decreased effectiveness of opioid-containing medications (e.g., cough syrups, antidiarrheals, opioid analgesics)

Drug Interactions

Naltrexone antagonizes the effects of opioid-containing medicines, such as cough and cold remedies, antidiarrheal preparations, and opioid analgesics.

Tests

LFTs, eosinophils, platelet count

METHADONE

Chemical Group
3-Heptan-1, 6-dimethylamino-4,4-diphenyl hydrochloride

Trade Name
Dolophine (Abbott)

Forms Available
Tablet: 5 and 10 mg; disket: 40 mg; injection: 10 mg per mL

Pharmacokinetics
Plasma half-life is 15 hours; peak plasma level in 4 hours

Dispensing
Divided daily doses as needed

Range of Dosing
Adults: For severe pain, 2.5 to 10 mg every 3 to 4 hours as needed
For detoxification treatment: Initially, 15 to 40 mg once daily for
   3 days; then decrease to q.i.d. or q.o.d. Higher doses may be
   needed for more severe physical dependence. Amount should
   always be enough to control withdrawal symptoms. Treatment duration longer than 21 days indicates progression from
   detoxification to maintenance treatment. Maintenance amount
   varies; maximum is 120 mg per day.
Children: not advised for patients younger than 18 years
Elderly: should be started on lower doses

FDA Approval
Detoxification (treatment of withdrawal syndrome) from opiate
addiction, severe pain

Possible Mechanism of Action
Acts at CNS mu opiate receptor agonist, mimicking the action
of morphine, suppressing the opiate withdrawal symptoms, and
responsible for analgesic effect

Possible Advantages
• Less addiction potential
• Long-acting agent
• Does not cause euphoria

Side Effects
• Respiratory depression
• Hypotension
• Dizziness and light-headedness
• Nausea and vomiting
• Sweating
• Sedation, dysphoria, and euphoria
• Constipation and urinary retention
• Decreased libido

Metabolism and Drug Interactions

Metabolized mainly by CYP 2B6 to metabolites 2-ethyl-5-methyl-3,3-diphenylpyrroline and 2-ethylidene-1,5-dimethyl-3,3-diphenylpyrrolidine, which are excreted in urine. Alteration of methadone levels can occur when combined with rifampin, phenothiazines, other narcotic analgesics, and CNS depressants.

Caution

Hepatic or renal impairment, hypothyroidism, addison disease, prostatic hypertrophy, urethral strictures, asthma, cor pulmonale, head injury; not advised for use in pregnancy, during lactation, and in patients younger than 18 years

BUPRENORPHINE

Chemical Group
Thebaine derivative

Trade Name
Buprenex (Reckitt-Benckiser)

Forms Available
Injection: 1 mL (0.3 mg of buprenorphine)

Pharmacokinetics
Half-life is 1.2 to 7.2 hours (mean ~2.2 hours); peak effect in 1 hour; effect lasts for 6 hours

Dispensing
Q.i.d. as needed

Range of Dosing
Adults: 1 mL (0.3 mg buprenorphine) IM or slow IV injection every 6 hours as needed; same 1-mL dose may be given 30 to 60 minutes after initial dose, if needed. In severe pain, 2 mL (0.6 mg buprenorphine) IM injection in a single dose may be given, providing stable patient response.
Children: 2 to 12 years: 2 to 6 μg per kg body weight every 4 to 6 hours as needed; not used in children younger than 2 years; never give repeat dose as in adults
Elderly: start on lower dose of 0.5 mL (1.5 mg buprenorphine)

FDA Approval
Relief of severe to moderate pain, treatment of opioid withdrawal

Possible Mechanism of Action
Acts on mu opiate receptors in the CNS as a partial agonist. High affinity and slow dissociation from receptors prevents exogenous opioids (e.g., heroin, morphine) from exerting strong agonist effects.

Possible Advantages
• Safe in patients younger than 18 years
• No dependence
• Does not produce euphoria
• Diminishes cravings

Side Effects
• Sedation
• Nausea and vomiting
• Dizziness/vertigo
• Sweating
• Respiratory depression
• Hypotension
• Miosis
• Headache
• Impaired fertility in rats

Metabolism and Drug Interactions

Metabolized by the hepatic CYP 3A4 isoenzyme and excreted in urine. CYP 3A4 inhibitors (e.g., erythromycin, ketoconazole, protease inhibitors) can elevate buprenorphine levels. CYP 3A4 inducers (e.g., rifampin, CBZ, phenytoin) can decrease buprenorphine levels. CNS depressants, MAOI, and other opioid narcotics can cause an exaggerated response when coadministered with buprenorphine.

Caution

Severe hepatic, renal, or pulmonary impairment; Addison's disease; prostatic hypertrophy; urethral strictures; hypothyroidism; CNS depression; acute alcoholism

DISULFIRAM

Chemical Group
bis(diethylthiocarbamoyl) disulfide

Trade Name
Antabuse (Sidmak)

Forms Available
Tablets: 250 and 500 mg

Pharmacokinetics
Half-life is approximately 10 hours, but enzyme-inhibiting effect can last longer (i.e., up to 14 days after discontinuation). Peak plasma level in 4 hours; peak enzyme-inhibiting effect reached after 3 daily doses

Dispensing
QD

Range of Dosing
Adults: initial dosing is a maximum of 500 mg daily, given in a single dose for 1 to 2 weeks. To minimize sedative effect, dose may be decreased. Never administer in acute alcohol intoxication. Average maintenance dose is 250 mg daily; range is 125 to 500 mg.
Children: not used
Elderly: start at low end of dosing range; continue therapy until sustained self-control has been established.

FDA Approval
Alcohol dependence

Possible Mechanism of Action
Aversive clinical reaction that occurs with consumption of alcohol, due to the accumulation of acetaldehyde, makes disulfiram a deterrent to alcohol use. Use only in motivated and compliant patients as an adjunct to other supportive and psychotherapeutic interventions.

Possible Advantages
Only preparation available for alcohol abuse

Side Effects
- Polyneuritis, peripheral neuropathy, optic neuritis
- Psychosis (including manic episodes) with higher doses or due to combined toxicity with metronidazole or isoniazid
- In first 2 weeks of therapy: fatigue, transient sedation, headache, acneiform eruption, allergic dermatitis, garlic or metallic aftertaste
- Hepatitis and hepatic necrosis

Metabolism and Drug Interactions

Metabolized in the liver to active metabolite diethylthiocarbaminic acid methyl ester; excreted in urine and expired as carbon disulfide

- Disulfiram–alcohol reaction: Inhibition of enzyme aldehyde dehydrogenase by disulfiram causes accumulation of acetaldehyde in the body, following ingestion of alcohol. Within 10 minutes, the high level of acetaldehyde causes symptoms such as facial flushing, headaches, sweating, nausea, vomiting, chest pain, blurred vision, dizziness, and confusion. In severe reactions, respiratory depression, arrhythmias, shock, seizures, or death may occur. Intensity of reaction depends on amount of alcohol and disulfiram taken. Reaction lasts as long as alcohol is present in blood; may last up to several hours.
- Disulfiram decreases metabolism and raises blood levels of metronidazole, isoniazid, phenytoin, diazepam, and oral anticoagulants. Adjust doses accordingly.

Caution

Diabetes mellitus, hypothyroidism, epilepsy, cerebral damage, nephritis, hepatic cirrhosis

Contraindications

- Acute alcohol intoxication
- Myocardial disease; coronary occlusion
- Psychosis
- Rubber contact dermatitis (hypersensitivity to thiuram derivatives)
- Nursing mothers
- Alcohol-containing preparations, such as cough syrups, vinegar, aftershave lotions, tonics

Tests

Baseline and follow-up LFTs, CBC, serum chemistries

ACAMPROSATE

Chemical Group
Calcium 3-acetylaminopropane-1-sulfonate

Trade Name
Campral (Merck KGaA)

Forms
Tablet: 333 mg

Pharmacokinetics
Absorption is via paracellular route in the GIT. Bioavailability decreases with food. Moderate distribution volume. Not protein bound. Steady-state plasma concentration after t.i.d dosing of 2 × 333-mg tablets in 3 to 8 hours.

Dispensing
T.i.d

Range of dosing
Adults: 2 tablets three times a day, for a total of 6 tablets a day; may lower dose as needed
Children: safety and effectiveness have not been studied.
Elderly: same as in adults; need dose adjustment in elderly with age-related kidney changes

FDA Approval
Alcohol dependence

Possible Mechanism of Action
Blocking glutaminergic N-methyl-D-aspartate receptors, while activating the $GABA_A$ receptors

Side Effects
- GI: diarrhea, nausea and vomiting, flatulence, stomach pain, loss of appetite, constipation, dry mouth
- Neurologic: headache, dizziness, drowsiness, insomnia, suicidal
- Cardiovascular: irregular pulse, irregular heartbeat, heart failure, sudden death
- Genitourinary: change in sexual desire or decrease in sexual ability, kidney failure
- Musculoskeletal: muscle/joint pain, backache, weight loss/gain
- Serious allergic reaction: itching, rash, swelling; burning and tingling of hands, feet, arms, or legs; trouble breathing

Contraindications
Hypersensitivity

Metabolism
Does not undergo metabolism. After oral dosing of 2 × 333 mg, the terminal half-life ranges from approximately 20 to 33 hours. Major route of excretion is via the kidneys as acamprosate.

Drug Interactions

Does not appear to interact with other medications often used during alcoholism treatment, such as disulfiram (Antabuse) and naltrexone (Revia), or with antianxiety, antidepressant, or hypnotic (sleep-inducing) medications

VARENICLINE

Chemical Group
7,8,9,10-tetrahydro-6,10-methano-6H-pyrazino[2,3-h][3]benzaze-pine, (2R,3R)-2,3-dihydroxybutanedioate (1:1)

Trade Name
Chantix (Pfizer)

Forms
0.5-mg and 1-mg capsular tablets

Pharmacokinetics
Maximum plasma concentrations occur within 3 to 4 hours after oral administration. Following administration of multiple oral doses, steady-state conditions were reached within 4 days.

Dispensing
0.5 mg once a day for 3 days, then 0.5 mg b.i.d. for 4 days, followed by 1 mg twice daily. It should be taken after eating and with a full glass of water. Patients should be treated for 12 weeks. For patients who have successfully stopped smoking at the end of 12 weeks, an additional course of 12-weeks treatment is recommended to further increase the likelihood of long-term abstinence.

FDA Approval
Smoking cessation

Possible Mechanism of Action
It binds with high affinity and selectivity at $\alpha_4\beta_2$ neuronal nicotinic acetylcholine receptors. The efficacy in smoking cessation is believed to be the result of varenicline's activity at a subtype of the nicotinic receptor where its binding produces agonist activity while simultaneously preventing nicotine binding to $\alpha_4\beta_2$ receptors.

Side Effects
The most common adverse events associated with it were nausea, sleep disturbance, constipation, flatulence, and vomiting.

Contraindications
None apparent

Metabolism
The elimination half-life is approximately 24 hours. It undergoes minimal metabolism with 92% excreted unchanged in the urine.

Drug Interactions
Cimetidine: Coadministration of cimetidine (300 mg q.i.d.), increased the systemic exposure of varenicline.

Nicotine replacement therapy (NRT): Coadministration of varenicline (1 mg b.i.d.) and transdermal nicotine (21 mg per day) for up to 12 days caused nausea, headache, vomiting, dizziness, dyspepsia, and fatigue.

Tests

Baseline and follow-up LFTs, RFT, CBC, serum chemistries. (See also bupropion [Zyban™].)

Cholinesterase Inhibitors and Related Drugs for the Elderly

DONEPEZIL

Chemical Group
Piperidine derivative

Trade Name
Aricept (Pfizer)

Forms Available
Tablet: 5 and 10 mg

Pharmacokinetics
Half-life is 70 hours; peak plasma level in 3 to 4 hours; steady state reached in 15 days

Dispensing
QD

Range of Dosing
Initial dose is 5 mg per day for 1 to 4 weeks; then increase to 10 mg per day if drug is tolerated. Range is 5 to 10 mg. Increased incidence of adverse effects with 10 mg dosing as compared with 5 mg.

FDA Approval
Mild to moderate dementia of Alzheimer's type

Possible Mechanism of Action
Reversible acetylcholinesterase inhibitor

Possible Advantages
- Once per day dosing
- Improved cognitive function on the ADAS-cog for as long as functioning cholinergic neurons remain intact; no alteration in actual disease process
- Has fewer side effects and is better tolerated than other cholinesterase inhibitors (e.g., rivastigmine, galantamine)
- Possible benefit in treatment of Down's syndrome

Side Effects
These are due to cholinergic effects and usually resolve spontaneously.
- Nausea
- Diarrhea
- Insomnia
- Fatigue
- Vomiting
- Muscle cramps

- Anorexia
- Bradycardia

Metabolism and Drug Interactions

Metabolized in the liver by CYP 3A3/4 and CYP 2D6; primarily excreted in the urine. Drugs that inhibit the CYP 3A4 and CYP 2D6 enzymes (e.g., ketoconazole and quinidine) can inhibit metabolism of donepezil and increase levels. Inducers of these enzymes (e.g., phenytoin, CBZ, dexamethasone, rifampin, phenobarbital) can increase metabolism of donepezil and lower the plasma levels.

Caution

Coadministration with other cholinergic agonists can potentiate vagal effects such as bradycardia, gastric acid secretion, and bladder outflow obstruction. Use in pregnancy with caution, due to possible teratogenic effect.

Tests

Heart rate monitoring before treatment; close observation recommended in patients with cardiac conduction delays or who are on beta-blockers

RIVASTIGMINE

Chemical Group

Carbamate derivative

Trade Name

Exelon (Novartis)

Forms Available

Capsule: 1.5, 3, 4.5, and 6 mg

Pharmacokinetics

Half-life is 1.5 hours; peak plasma level reached in 1 hour. Doubling the dose from 6 to 12 mg may cause a threefold increase in blood levels due to nonlinear elimination kinetics at a higher dosing range. Clearance may decrease by more than 60% in patients with hepatic or renal impairment.

Dispensing

B.i.d. with meals in morning and evening

Range of Dosing

Initially, 1.5 mg b.i.d. may increase dose by 1.5 mg every 2 weeks provided patient is tolerant of adverse effects. Range is 6 to 12 mg per day.

FDA Approval

Mild to moderate dementia of Alzheimer's type and associated with Parkinson's disease

Possible Mechanism of Action

Reversible selective cholinesterase inhibitor

Possible Advantages

- Limits cognitive decline in patients with moderate disease
- More efficient than galantamine and donepezil in treating advanced stages of dementia due to nonselective inhibition of both acetylcholinesterase and butyrylcholinesterase activity which is more predominant in advanced stages of dementia
- Effective in treating Lewy body dementia

Side Effects

Least tolerated of the cholinesterase inhibitors. Excessive central nervous selectivity causes increased amount of nausea and vomiting. Side effects are due to cholinergic activity, including:

- Nausea and vomiting
- Diarrhea
- Anorexia
- Dizziness
- Headache
- Bradycardia
- Abdominal pain
- Fatigue

Metabolism and Drug Interactions

Metabolized by cholinesterase-mediated hydrolysis at site of target enzyme and excreted in urine; for this reason, drugs that are metabolized by the P450 isoenzymes do not interact with rivastigmine

Caution

Due to cholinomimetic action, use with caution in cardiac conduction disorders, with drugs that cause bradycardia, in patients prone to ulcer disease or GI bleeding, and in asthmatics. Not recommended in pregnancy due to possible teratogenic effect; contraindicated in severe renal or hepatic impairment

Tests

Heart rate monitoring before treatment; close observation recommended in patients with cardiac conduction delays or who are on beta-blockers

GALANTAMINE

Chemical Group
(4aS,6R,8aS)-4a,5,9,10,11,12-hexahydro-3-methoxy-11-methyl-6 H—benzofuro [3a, 3, 2ef] [2] benzazepin—6—ol hydrobromide

Trade Name
Razadyne (Janssen)

Forms Available
Tablet: 4, 8, and 12 mg; oral solution (4 mg per mL) in 100-mL bottle

Pharmacokinetics
Half-life of 7 hours; peak plasma level reached in 1 hour. Oral bioavailability is 90% for both oral solution and tablet forms.

Dispensing
B.i.d. or t.i.d. taken with meals

Range of Dosing
Initially, 4 mg b.i.d.; if well tolerated, increase dose to 8 mg b.i.d. after 4 weeks. Further increase dose after 4 additional weeks to 12 mg b.i.d. (or 8 mg t.i.d.), if needed. Range is 8 to 24 mg per day. In patients with moderate hepatic or renal impairment, dose should not exceed 16 mg per day.

FDA Approval
Mild to moderate dementia of Alzheimer's type

Possible Mechanism of Action
Reversible, competitive acetylcholinesterase inhibitor

Possible Advantages
- Mini-Mental State Examination score improvements greatest compared with other cholinesterase inhibitors
- Potential role in treatment of vascular dementia

Side Effects
Due to cholinergic effects and usually resolve in 5 to 7 days:
- Nausea
- Vomiting
- Diarrhea
- Anorexia and weight loss
- Headache
- Bradycardia and AV block
- Fatigue

Metabolism and Drug Interaction
Metabolized in the liver by isoenzymes CYP 2D6 and CYP 3A4; excreted in urine. Concentrations increase with coadministration of drugs that inhibit these enzymes, such as paroxetine and ketoconazole. Severe renal impairment reduces the clearance of galantamine up to 66%.

Caution

Due to cholinomimetic action, use with caution in cardiac conduction disorders, with drugs that cause bradycardia, and in patients prone to ulcer disease or GI bleeding and in asthmatics. Not recommended in pregnancy due to possible teratogenic effect; contraindicated in severe renal or hepatic impairment

Tests

Heart rate monitoring before treatment; close observation recommended in patients with cardiac conduction delays or who are on beta-blockers

MEMANTINE

Chemical Group
1-Amino-3,5-dimethyladamantane hydrochloride

Trade Name
Namenda (Forest)

Forms Available
Tablet: 5 and 10 mg; titration packs include 28×5 mg and 21×10 mg tablets

Pharmacokinetics
Half-life of 60 to 80 hours; peak levels reached in 3 to 7 hours. Clearance is reduced with alkaline urine.

Dispensing
Once daily to start, then b.i.d.

Range of Dosing
Initially, 5 mg once daily. Dose is increased by 5-mg increments in at least 1-week intervals to 10 mg per day (5 mg b.i.d.), 15 mg per day (5 and 10 mg as separate doses), and finally 20 mg per day (10 mg b.i.d.). Target dose is 20 mg per day. Dose should be lowered in moderate renal impairment. Use in severe renal impairment is not recommended.

FDA Approval
Moderate to severe dementia of Alzheimer's type

Possible Mechanism of Action
N-methyl-D-aspartate receptor antagonist; provides neuroprotection by blocking glutamate excitotoxicity in brain, preventing calcium buildup

Possible Advantages
- May be used in combination with cholinesterase inhibitors due to different mechanism of action
- Improves activities of daily living, social behavior, and lack of drive, as well as cognitive function
- Possible benefit in treatment of chronic pain, drug cravings, dementia in AIDS, multiple sclerosis, and glaucoma is being researched.

Side Effects
- Frequent: confusion, dizziness, headache, fatigue, hallucination
- Infrequent: anxiety, hypertonus, vomiting, bladder infection, increased sex drive

Metabolism and Drug Interactions
Majority (57% to 82%) of memantine is not metabolized and is excreted unchanged in the urine. The remaining portion is metabolized to inactive metabolites in the liver. Drug is not metabolized through the P450 enzyme system. Levels may increase with

coadministration of drugs that alkalinize urine (e.g., carbonic an-hydrase inhibitors, sodium bicarbonate). Drug interactions may also occur with drugs that undergo elimination by the same renal mechanism (e.g., hydrochlorothiazide, triamterene, cimetidine, ranitidine, guanidine).

Contraindications

Severe renal or hepatic impairment, pregnancy, hypersensitivity to memantine

Caution

Conditions with raised urinary pH

Miscellaneous Medications

PROPRANOLOL

Chemical Group
1-(Isopropylamino)-3-(1-naphthyloxy)-2-propanol

Trade Name
Inderal (Wyeth-Ayerst)

Forms Available
Tablet: 10, 20, 40, 60, and 80 mg; long-acting tablet: 60, 80, 120, and 160 mg; injectable: 1 mg per mL

Pharmacokinetics
Half-life approximately 4 hours; peak effect in 1 to 1.5 hours

Dispensing
B.i.d. or t.i.d.

Range of Dosing
Adults: 10 to 120 mg per day
Children: usually 2 to 8 mg per kg per day, up to three times per day
Elderly: no specific dose range has been established for psychotropic use.

FDA Approval
- Management of hypertension
- Long-term treatment of angina pectoris
- Supraventricular arrhythmias: paroxysmal atrial tachycardia, Wolff–Parkinson–White syndrome, persistent sinus tachycardia, thyrotoxic arrhythmias, persistent atrial extrasystoles, atrial flutter and fibrillation
- Ventricular tachycardia that is not caused by catecholamines or digitalis

Possible Mechanism of Action
Nonselective, beta-adrenergic receptor blocker agent

Possible Advantages
- Drug of choice for akathisia
- Commonly used in psychiatry for reducing arousal and agitation: Tourette's syndrome, ADHD, aggression, self-abuse

Side Effects
- CV: hypotension, bradycardia
- CNS: mental depression, light-headedness, amnesia, emotional liability, confusion, hallucinations, dizziness, fatigue, insomnia, hypersomnolence, psychosis, cognitive dysfunction
- Skin: rash, alopecia, exfoliative dermatitis, hyperkeratosis

- Endocrine system: hypoglycemia or hyperglycemia, lipid abnormalities, hyperkalemia
- GIT: diarrhea, nausea, vomiting, stomach discomfort, constipation, anorexia
- Hematology: agranulocytosis, thrombocytopenia
- Respiratory system: wheezing, bronchospasm, pulmonary edema
- Ocular: mydriasis, decreased production of tears, hyperemia of conjunctiva, decreased visual acuity

Metabolism and Drug Interactions

Extensive first-pass metabolism; metabolized in liver by CYP 12A, 2C18, and 2D6 into active and inactive compounds; blunted effect with nonspecific beta-agonists. Concurrent use with alpha-blocker increases risk of orthostasis.

Caution

Diabetes, glaucoma, thyrotoxicosis

Contraindications

Bronchial asthma, congestive heart failure, cardiogenic shock, sinus bradycardia, and greater than first-degree heart block

DESMOPRESSIN

Chemical Group
Synthetic analogue of natural antidiuretic hormone (D-arginine vasopressin monoacetate trihydrate)

Trade Name
DDAVP (Rhone-Poulenc Rorer)

Forms Available
Tablet: 0.1 and 0.2 mg; nasal spray: 100 μg per mL nasal

Pharmacokinetics
Half-life is 75 minutes; onset of action in 1 hour with peak effect seen in 1 to 5 hours; duration of action is 5 to 21 hours

Dispensing
QHS

Range of Dosing
Children: age 6 years or older for nocturnal enuresis: initial dosage of 0.2 mg (0.2 mL) at bedtime; half dose is given in each nostril. Range is 0.1 to 0.4 mg.
Elderly: no information available

FDA Approval
Primary nocturnal enuresis, central diabetes insipidus

Possible Mechanism of Action
Like the naturally occurring hormone, DDAVP binds to vaso-pressin (V2) receptor sites in the collecting ducts of the kidneys, thus increasing the cellular permeability of the collecting duct to H_2O. By enhancing reabsorption, DDAVP achieves an antidiuretic effect, decreasing urine volume and increasing urine concentration (osmolality).

Possible Advantages
DDAVP is used for enuresis.

Side Effects
1% to 10%: facial flushing, headache, dizziness, nausea, abdominal cramps, nasal congestion
Less than 1%: hyponatremia, elevated blood pressure, water intoxication

Metabolism and Drug Interactions
Metabolism is unknown. Demeclocycline and lithium may decrease ADH effect. Chlorpropamide and fludrocortisone may increase ADH effect.

Tests
Periodic sodium levels

Medication Clinic Progress Note Format

Vital Signs

Blood pressure, pulse, weight, and height

Target Symptoms (index/present)

Intervention-Effect (present/future-reasoning)

- Biological:

  -Medication
  -Effect
  -Side effects
  -Patient education (what, why, when, how much)

- Psychological
- Social
- School/work
- Liaison with other agencies involved

Risk of Tardive Dyskinesia

Explained where relevant—Yes/NA

B. Lithium Laboratory Monitoring

Patient's name _____   Height _____

Date	Ratings		For months of lithium and dose	No. of hours since last dose	Test (frequency)								
	Depression 0–6	Mania 0–6			Serum lithium (q2mo + prn)	Serum creatinine (q6mo)	Urine-specific gravity (q6mo)	24-Hr urine volume (q6mo)	T$_4$RIA (q1y)	T$_3$RU (q1y)	TSH (q1y)	Weight (q1y)

Frequency of monitoring depends on many factors and may be done more or less often. Stable patients are usually monitored less often. T$_4$RIA = serum T$_4$ by radioimmunoassay; T$_3$RU = tri-iodothyrorine resin uptake; TSH = thyroid stimulating hormone

C Abnormal Involuntary Movement Scale—Modified (AIMS-M3D)

Patient's name _____   Date _____   Medications _____

Code: 0 = none; 1 = minimal, maybe extreme normal; 2 = mild; 3 = moderate; 4 = severe (ratings for maximum movement during rating period);
A = movement present only during activation; NR = not ratable.

| Body Region | Tardive Dyskinesialike Movements | | | | | Nontardive Dyskinesialike Movements | | | |
	Not Ratable	Abnormal (yes/no)?	Choreo-athetosis	Dystonia	Movement Type (Circle if appropriate)	Tic*	Mannerism/ stereotypy	Tremor	Other (specify)
1. Muscles of facial expression	NR	Y/N	0 1 2 3 4 A	0 1 2 3 4	Movements of forehead, eyebrows, or periorbital area; include frowning, blinking**	0 1 2 3 4	0 1 2 3 4	0 1 2 3 4	0 1 2 3 4
2. Lips and perioral region	NR	Y/N	0 1 2 3 4 A	0 1 2 3 4	Puckering, pouting, smacking, cheeks puff out	0 1 2 3 4	0 1 2 3 4	0 1 2 3 4	0 1 2 3 4
3. Jaw	NR	Y/N	0 1 2 3 4 A	0 1 2 3 4	Biting, clenching, chewing, mouth opening	0 1 2 3 4	0 1 2 3 4	0 1 2 3 4	0 1 2 3 4
4. Tongue	NR	Y/N	0 1 2 3 4 A	0 1 2 3 4	Movements only in and out of mouth	0 1 2 3 4	0 1 2 3 4	0 1 2 3 4	0 1 2 3 4
5. Upper extremities	NR	Y/N	R. 0 1 2 3 4 A L. 0 1 2 3 4 A	0 1 2 3 4	Arm, wrist, hand, fingers Arm, wrist, hand, fingers	0 1 2 3 4	0 1 2 3 4	0 1 2 3 4	0 1 2 3 4
						0 1 2 3 4	0 1 2 3 4	0 1 2 3 4	0 1 2 3 4

(continued)

C Abnormal Involuntary Movement Scale—Modified (AIMS-M3D) (Continued)

	Tardive Dyskinesialike Movements					Nontardive Dyskinesialike Movements			
Body Region	**Not Ratable**	**Abnormal (yes/no)?**	**Choreo-athetosis**	**Dystonia**	**Movement Type (Circle if appropriate)**	**Tic***	**Mannerism/ stereotypy**	**Tremor**	**Other (specify)**
6. Lower extremities	NR	R. Y/N L.	R. 0 1 2 3 4 A L. 0 1 2 3 4 A	0 1 2 3 4 0 1 2 3 4	Legs, knees, ankles, toes, lateral knee movement, foot tapping, heel dropping, foot squirming, inversion and eversion of foot	0 1 2 3 4 0 1 2 3 4	0 1 2 3 4 0 1 2 3 4	0 1 2 3 4 0 1 2 3 4	0 1 2 3 4 0 1 2 3 4
7. Trunk	NR	Y/N	0 1 2 3 4 A	0 1 2 3 4	Neck, shoulders, hips, rocking, twisting, pelvic gyrations, diaphragm	0 1 2 3 4	0 1 2 3 4	0 1 2 3 4	0 1 2 3 4

General Tardive Dyskinesia-like Rating Items (1–7) 0 1 2 3 4	*Tics may occasionally be part of tardive dyskinesia. **Increased blinking may be part of a psychotic illness.	8. Bradykinesia (Y/N)? R. 0 1 2 3 4 L. 0 1 2 3 4	9. Rigidity (Y/N)? R. 0 1 2 3 4 L. 0 1 2 3 4	10. Loss of facial expression 0 1 2 3 4	11. Abnormal gait and posture 0 1 2 3 4	12. Akathisia 0 1 2 3 4		
Patient awareness 0 1 2 3 4 Incapacitation 0 1 2 3 4	Problems with teeth/dentures (Y/N)? If "yes," what kind?	Date: Previous Total AIMS Scores:						

TOTAL Tardive Dyskinesia-like Score (1–7)
(use average of both sides for items 5 and 6)
Choreoathetosis   Dystonia

D Pediatric Side Effects Checklist (P-SEC)

This Checklist is to be completed by parent, child, or patient. This will help to identify the adverse effects of the medications. Please read through the list and check ( ) in the appropriate box.

| Patient Name: | | Id: | | Date: | |

PROBLEMS	NONE	MILD/INTERFERES SOMETIMES BUT TOLERABLE	MODERATE/ INTERFERES SOMEWHAT	SEVERE/ INTERFERES A LOT
Gastrointestinal system				
Discomfort in the stomach				
Constipation				
Diarrhea				
Increased appetite				
Decreased appetite				
Nausea/Vomiting				
Central Nervous system				
Muscle trembling/Shaking				
Sleepiness				
Difficulty falling asleep				
Muscle stiffness				
Stiff jaw				

(continued)

D Pediatric Side Effects Checklist (P-SEC) (*Continued*)

PROBLEMS	NONE	MILD/INTERFERES SOMETIMES BUT TOLERABLE	MODERATE/ INTERFERES SOMEWHAT	SEVERE/ INTERFERES A LOT
Problem concentrating				
Problems with memory				
Restlessness/wanting to pace				
Irritable/agitated				
Problems with speech				
Dizziness/light-headedness				
Headache				
Seizures				
Nightmares/vivid dreams				
Blurring of vision				
Excessive drooling				
Increased sweating				
Dry mouth/eyes				
Skin				
Rash				
Acne				
Hair loss				

Cardiovascular system							
Palpitations							
Blackouts/loss of consciousness							
Chest pain							
Endocrine system							
Feeling cold /hot							
Weight gain							
Weight loss							
Fatigue/tiredness							
Breast cyst							
Changes in menstrual periods							
Mood/behavior changes							
Depression/feeling sad							
Excitable							
Feeling anxious							
Aggressive							
Panic attacks							
Renal system							
Increased urination							
Bed wetting							
Frothy urine/red colored urine							
Sexual concerns/problems							

(continued)

D Pediatric Side Effects Checklist (P-SEC) (*Continued*)

> ## Please indicate your current medications here

MEDICATION	Dose

This checklist (P-SEC) accounts for most of the possible side effects seen with medications utilized in psychopharmacotherapy.
For comments, e-mail: mpavuluri@psych.uic.edu

E

Abbreviations

A
A, Adrenergic
ACE, Angiotensis-converting enzyme
ADAS, Alzheimer's disease assessment scale
ADH, Antidiuretic hormone
ADHD, Attention-deficit hyperactivity disorder
ANS, Autonomic nervous system
AUC, Area under the curve
AV, Atrioventricular

B
b.i.d., Twice a day
BUN, Blood urea nitrogen
BZD, Benzodiazepine

C
cAMP, Cyclic adenosine monophosphate
CBC, Complete blood cell count
CBZ, Carbamazepine
CD, Controlled delivery
C_{max}, Maximum concentration
CMP, Complete metabolic profile
CNS, Central nervous system
CR, Controlled release
CVS, Cardiovascular system
CYP, Cytochrome P

D
D, Dopamine
DA, Dopamine and adrenergic
DARI, Dopamine and adrenergic reuptake inhibitor
DKA, Diabetic ketoacidosis
DRI, Dopamine reuptake inhibitor

E
ECG, Electrocardiogram
EEG, Electroencephalogram
EPS, Extrapyramidal symptoms
ER, Extended release
ESR, Erythrocyte sedimentation rate

F
FDA, Food and Drug Administration
FGA, First-generation antipsychotics

G
GABA, Gamma-aminobutyric acid
GAD, General anxiety disorder
GFR, Glomerular filtration rate

GGT, Gamma glutamyl transferase
GI, Gastrointestinal
GIT, Gastrointestinal tract

H
HCA, Heterocyclic
HCG, Human chorionic gonadotropin
HIV, Human immunodeficiency virus

I
IM, Intramuscular
IR, Immediate release
IV, Intravenous

L
LFT, Liver function test

M
MAOI, Monoamine oxidase inhibitor
MDD, Major depressive disorder
MHD, 10-Monohydroxy metabolite
MI, Myocardial infarction

N
NaSSA, Noradrenergic and specific serotonergic antagonist
NE, Norepinephrine
NRI, Norepinephrine reuptake inhibitor
NSAID, Nonsteroidal anti-inflammatory drug

O
OCD, Obsessive-compulsive disorder

P
PCOS, Polycystic ovarian syndrome
PIP, Phosphoinositol phosphate
PKC, Protein kinase C
PLG, Polylactide-co-glycolide
PMDD, Premenstrual dysphoric disorder
PMNL, Polymorphonuclear leukocytes
PTSD, Posttraumatic stress disorder

Q
QHS, Every hour
q.i.d., Four times a day

R
REM, Rapid eye movement
RFT, Renal function test

S
SARI, Serotonin-adrenergic reuptake inhibitor
S-CT, S-enantiomer of citalopram
SGPT, Serum glutamate pyruvate transferase

SIADH, Syndrome of inappropriate antidiuretic hormone
SNRI, Serotonin and norepinephrine reuptake inhibitor
SR, Sustained release
SRI, Serotonin reuptake inhibitor
SSRI, Selective serotonin reuptake inhibitor

T
T_3, Thyroxine
T_4, Thyronine
TFT, Thyroid function test
t.i.d., Three times a day
T_{max}, Time to maximum concentration
TSH, Thyroid-stimulating hormone

U
UTI, Urinary tract infection

W
WBC, White blood (cell) count

X
XR, Extended release

REFERENCE

Janicak PG, Davis JM, Perskorn SH, et al. *Principles and Practice of Psychopharmacotherapy.* 4th ed. Philadelphia: Lippincott Williams & Wilkins; 2006.

Index

Page numbers followed by f indicate figure; those followed by t indicate table.

A

Abbreviations, 151–153
Abilify (aripiprazole), 21–22
Abnormal involuntary movement scale—modified (AIMS-M3D), 145–146
Acamprosate, 127–128
Acetamide hydrochloride (guanfacine), 91–92
Adderall (dextroamphetamine sulfate and amphetamine sulfate), 105–106, 113t
Adjuvant medications, 89–92
  clonidine, 89–90
  guanfacine, 91–92
AIMS-M3D (abnormal involuntary movement scale—modified), 145–146
Alprazolam (benzodiazepines), 73–75, 74t, 75t
Ambien (zolpidem), 81–82
1-Amino-3,5-dimethyladamantane hydrochloride (memantine), 137–138
2-Aminoethyl oxime ether of aralkylketone (fluvoxamine), 35–36
Aminoketone group (bupropion), 49–50
1-(Aminomethyl) cyclohexaneacetic acid (gabapentin), 65–66
Amitriptyline, 23–26, 24t. See also Antidepressants, first-generation
Amoxapine, 23–26, 24t. See also Antidepressants, first-generation
Antabuse (disulfiram), 125–126
Antidepressants, first-generation, 23–26
  available forms of, 23
  chemical groups and trade names of, 23, 24t
  dispensing and dosing of, 23, 24t
  drug interactions of, 26
  FDA approval of, 24
  mechanism of action of, 24
  pharmacokinetics of, 23
  possible advantages of, 24
  side effects of, 25t, 26
Antidepressants, second-generation, 27–52
  bupropion, 49–50
  citalopram, 37–38
  duloxetine, 51–52
  escitalopram, 39–40
  fluoxetine, 27–29
  fluvoxamine, 35–36
  mirtazapine, 47–48
  nefazodone, 43–44
  paroxetine, 33–34
  sertraline, 31–32
  trazodone, 45–46
  venlafaxine, 41–42
Antiepileptic agents, other, 63–72
  gabapentin, 65–66
  oxcarbazepine, 63–64
  tiagabine, 67
  topiramate, 69
  zonisamide, 71–72
Antipsychotics, first-generation, 1–5. See also specific agents
  advantages of, 1
  chlorpromazine, 2t
  drug interactions of, 5
  fluphenazine, 3t
  haloperidol, 2t
  loxapine, 4t
  mechanism of action of, 1, 5f (See also specific agents)
  mesoridazine, 3t
  molindone, 3t
  perphenazine, 4t
  pimozide, 4t
  side effects of, 1, 5, 5f
  thioridazine, 2t
  thiothixene, 4t
  trifluoperazine, 3t
Antipsychotics, second-generation, 6–22. See also specific agents
  aripiprazole, 21–22
  clozapine, 6–8
  olanzapine, 13–14

Antipsychotics (*Contd.*)
  paliperidone extended
    release, 11–12
  quetiapine, 15–16
  risperidone, 9–10
  ziprasidone, 17–19, 18f
Anxiolytics/sedative-hypnotics,
    73–88
  benzodiazepines, 73–75, 74t,
    75t
  buspirone, 77
  eszoplicone, 85–86
  pregabalin, 79
  ramelteon, 87–88
  zaleplon, 83–84
  zolpidem, 81–82
D-Arginine vasopressin
    monoacetate trihydrate
    (desmopressin), 141
Aricept (donepezil), 131–132
Aripiprazole, 21–22
Ascendin (amoxapine,
    clomipramine), 23–26, 24t.
    See also Antidepressants,
    first-generation
Atomoxetine, 109–110, 114t
Attentin (atomoxetine),
    109–110, 114t
Azaspirodecanedione
    (buspirone), 77

B

Benzenepropanamine,
    N-methyl-gamma-(2-
    methylphenoxy)-
    hydrochloride
    (atomoxetine), 109–110,
    114t
Benzisothiazole (ziprasidone),
    17–19, 18f
Benzisoxazole (risperidone),
    9–10
Benzisoxazole derivative
    (paliperidone extended
    release), 11–12
1-2-Benzisoxazole-3-
    methanesulfonamide
    (zonisamide), 71–72
Benzodiazepines, 73–75, 74t,
    75t, 154–155
Bis(diethylthiocarbamoyl)
    disulfide (disulfiram),
    125–126
Buprenex (buprenorphine),
    123–124

Buprenorphine, 123–124
Bupropion, 49–50
Buspar (buspirone), 77
Buspirone, 77

C

Calcium 3-acetylaminopropane-
    1-sulfonate (acamprosate),
    127–128
Campral (acamprosate), 127–128
Carbamate derivative
    (rivastigmine), 133–134
Carbamazepine, 61–62
Catapres (clonidine), 89–90
Celexa (citalopram), 37–38
Chantix (varenicline), 129–130
Chlorpromazine, 2t
Cholinerasterase inhibitors and
    related drugs for elderly,
    131–138
  donepezil, 131–132
  galantamine, 135–136
  memantine, 137–138
  rivastigmine, 133–134
Choreoathetosis, AIMS-M3D
    for, 145–146
Citalopram, 37–38
Clomipramine, 23–26, 24t.
    See also Antidepressants,
    first-generation
Clonazepam (benzodiazepines),
    73–75, 74t, 75t
Clonidine, 89–90
Clozapine, 6–8
Clozaril (clozapine), 6–8
Concerta, extended release
    (methylphenidate), 95–96,
    114t. *See also*
    Methylphenidate (HCl)
Cylert (methylphenidate HCl),
    114t
Cymbalta (duloxetine), 51–52

D

Daytrana (methylphenidate,
    transdermal system),
    97–98, 114t
DDAVP (desmopressin), 141
Depacone (valproate), 57–58
Depacote (valproate), 57–58
Depakene (valproate), 57–58
Desipramine, 23–26, 24t.
    See also Antidepressants,
    first-generation
Desmopressin, 141

Desyrel (trazodone), 23–26, 24t,
    45–46. *See also*
    Antidepressants,
    first-generation
Dexedrine
    (dextroamphetamine),
    103–104, 113t
Dexmethylphenidate, 101–102,
    114t
Dextroamphetamine prodrug
    (lisdexamfetamine
    dimesylate), 111–112, 113t,
    115
Dextroamphetamine sulfate,
    103–104, 113t
Dextroamphetamine sulfate and
    amphetamine sulfate
    (Adderall), 105–106, 113t
DextroStat
    (dextroamphetamine),
    103–104, 113t
Diazepam (benzodiazepines),
    73–75, 74t, 75t
Dibenzodiazepines
    amoxapine, 23–26, 24t
    (*See also* Antidepressants,
    first-generation)
    clozapine, 6–8
Dibenzothiazepine (quetiapine),
    15–16
10,11-Dihydro-10-oxo-5-H
    dibenzapine-5 carboxamide
    (oxcarbazepine), 63–64
2-[(Diphenylmethyl)sulfinyl]
    acetamide (modafinil),
    107–108, 114t
Disulfiram, 125–126
Divalproex sodium (valproate),
    57–58
Dolophine (methadone),
    121–122
Donepezil, 131–132
Doxepin, 23–26, 24t. *See also*
    Antidepressants,
    first-generation
Duloxetine, 51–52
Dystonia, AIMS-M3D for,
    145–146

E
Effexor (venlafaxine), 41–42
Elavil (amitriptyline), 23–26,
    24t. *See also*
    Antidepressants,
    first-generation

Emsam (selegiline TS), 23–26,
    24t. *See also*
    Antidepressants,
    first-generation
Equetro (carbamazepine), 61–62
Escitalopram, 39–40
Eskalith (lithium), 53–56.
    See also Lithium
Eszoplicone, 85–86
Exelon (rivastigmine), 133–134

F
Fluoxetine, 27–29
Fluoxetine plus olanzapine
    (Symbyax), 154–155
Fluphenazine, 3t
Fluvoxamine, 35–36
Focalin (dexmethylphenidate),
    101–102, 114t

G
Gabapentin, 65–66
Gabitril (tiagabine), 67
Galantamine, 135–136
Geodon (ziprasidone), 17–19, 18f
Guanfacine, 91–92

H
Haldol (haloperidol), 2t
Haloperidol, 2t
5H-Dibenzapine-5-carboxamide
    (carbamazepine), 61–62
3-Heptan-1,6-dimethylamino-
    4,4-diphenyl hydrochloride
    (methadone), 121–122
Heterocyclic antidepressants
    (HCAs), 23–26
    available forms of, 23
    chemical groups and trade
        names of, 23, 24t
    dispensing and dosing of, 23,
        24t
    drug interactions of, 26
    FDA approval of, 24
    mechanism of action of, 24
    pharmacokinetics of, 23
    possible advantages of, 24
    side effects of, 25t, 26

I
Imidazoline (clonidine), 89–90
Imidazopyridine (zolpidem),
    81–82
Imipramine, 23–26, 24t.
    See also Antidepressants,
    first-generation

Inderal (propranolol), 139–140
Invega (paliperidone extended
  release), 11–12
1-(Isopropylamino)-3-(1-
  napthyloxy)-2-propanol
  (propranolol), 139–140

L
Lamictal (lamotrigine), 59–60
Lamotrigine, 59–60
Lexapro (escitalopram), 39–40
Lisdexamfetamine dimesylate,
  111–112, 113t, 115
Lithium, 53–56
  dispensing and dosing of, 53
  FDA approval of, 53
  mechanism of action of, 53
  metabolism and drug
    interactions of, 55
  pharmacokinetics of, 53
  possible advantages of,
    53–54
  side effects of, 54
  special groups of users of, 55
  tests of, 55–56
  toxicity of, 55
  trade names and available
    forms of, 53
  withdrawal effects of, 54–55
Lithium carbonate (lithium),
  53–56. *See also* Lithium
Lithium citrate syrup (lithium),
  53–56. *See also* Lithium
Lithium laboratory monitor,
  144
Lithobid (lithium), 53–56.
  See also Lithium
L-lysine-*d*-amphetamine
  (lisdexamfetamine
  dimesylate), 111–112, 113t,
  115
Long QT, from second-
  generation antipsychotics,
  17–18, 18f
Lorazepam (benzodiazepines),
  73–75, 74t, 75t
Loxapine, 4t
Loxitane (loxapine), 4t
Ludiomil (maprotiline),
  23–26, 24t. *See also*
  Antidepressants, first-
  generation
Lunesta (eszoplicone), 85–86
Luvox (fluvoxamine), 35–36
Lyrica (pregabalin), 79

M
Mannerism, AIMS-M3D for,
  145–146
Maprotiline, 23–26, 24t.
  See also Antidepressants,
  first-generation
Medication clinic progress note
  format, 143
Melatonin synthetic analog
  (ramelteon), 87–88
Mellaril (thioridazine), 2t
Memantine, 137–138
Mesoridazine, 3t
Metadate, controlled delivery
  (methylphenidate HCl),
  99–100, 114t
Methadone, 121–122
Methylin (methylphenidate
  HCl), 113t
2-Methyl-4-(4-methyl-1-
  piperazinyl)-10*H*-
  thieno[2,3-b] [1,5]
  benzodiazepine (Symbyax),
  154–155
Methylphenidate (HCl), 93–102
  Concerta, extended release,
    95–96, 114t
  Cylert, 114t
  dexmethylphenidate,
    101–102, 114t
  Metadate, 99–100, 114t
  Ritalin, 93–94, 113t
  transdermal system, 97–98,
    114t
Midazolam (benzodiazepines),
  73–75, 74t, 75t
Mirtazapine, 47–48
Moban (molindone), 3t
Modafinil, 107–108, 114t
Molindone, 3t
Monoamine oxidase inhibitors
  (MAOIs), 23–26
  available forms of, 23
  chemical groups and trade
    names of, 23, 24t
  dispensing and dosing of, 23,
    24t
  drug interactions of, 26
  FDA approval of, 24
  mechanism of action of, 24
  pharmacokinetics of, 23
  possible advantages of, 24
  side effects of, 25t, 26
Monovalent cation (lithium),
  53–56. *See also* Lithium

Mood stabilizers, 53–62. *See also*
   Antiepileptic agents, other
   carbamazepine, 61–62
   lamotrigine, 59–60
   lithium, 53–56 (*See also*
      Lithium)
   valproate, 57–58

N

Nalorex (naltrexone), 116–117
Naltrexone, 116–117
Naltrexone extended release,
   119–120
Namenda (memantine), 137–138
Nardil (phenelzine), 23–26, 24t.
   See also Antidepressants,
   first-generation
Navane (thiothixene), 4t
Nefazodone, 43–44
Neurontin (gabapentin), 65–66
N-methyl-3-phenyl-3-[α, α,
   α-(trifluoro-*p*-tolyl)-oxy]
   propylamine hydrochloride
   (fluoxetine), 27–28
Nontardive dyskinesialike
   movements, AIMS-M3D for,
   145–146
Norpramin (desipramine),
   23–26, 24t. *See also*
   Antidepressants,
   first-generation
Nortriptyline, 23–26, 24t.
   See also Antidepressants,
   first-generation
Note format, medication clinic
   progress, 143

O

Olanzapine, 13
Olanzapine plus fluoxetine
   (Symbyax), 14
Orap (pimozide), 4t
Oxazepam (benzodiazepines),
   73–75, 74t, 75t
Oxcarbazepine, 63–64
Oxymorphone congeners
   naltrexone, 116–117
   naltrexone extended release,
   119–120

P

Paliperidone extended release,
   11–12
Pamelor (nortriptyline),
   23–26, 24t. *See also*

Antidepressants, first-
   generation
Parnate (tranylcypromine),
   23–26, 24t. *See also*
   Antidepressants, first-
   generation
Paroxetine, 33–34
Paxil (paroxetine), 33–34
Pediatric side effect checklist
   (P-SEC), 147–150
Perphenazine, 4t
Phenelzine, 23–26, 24t. *See also*
   Antidepressants, first-
   generation
Phenethylamine bicyclic
   derivative (venlafaxine),
   41–42
Phenylpiperazines
   nefazodone, 43–44
   trazodone, 23–26, 24t
      (*See also* Antidepressants,
      first-generation)
Phenylpiperidine salt
   (paroxetine), 33–34
Phenyltriazine (lamotrigine),
   59–60
Phthalane derivatives
   citalopram, 37–38
   escitalopram, 39–40
Pimozide, 4t
Piperazino-azepine group
   (mirtazapine), 47–48
Piperidine derivatives
   donepezil, 131–132
   methylphenidate, 93–102,
   114t (*See also*
      Methylphenidate (HCl))
Pregabalin, 79
Prolixin (fluphenazine), 3t
Propranolol, 139–140
2-Propyl-pentanoic acid
   (valproate), 57–58
Protriptyline, 23–26, 24t.
   See also Antidepressants,
   first-generation
Provigil (modafinil), 107–108,
   114t
Prozac (fluoxetine), 27–29
P-SEC (pediatric side effect
   checklist), 147–150
Psychostimulants, 93–115,
   113t–114t
   Adderall (dextroamphetamine
   sulfate and amphetamine
   sulfate), 105–106, 113t

Psychostimulants (*Contd.*)
  atomoxetine, 109–110, 114t
  dextroamphetamine,
    103–104, 113t
  lisdexamfetamine dimesylate,
    111–112, 113t, 115
  methylphenidate, 93–102
    (*See also* Methylphenidate
    (HCl))
  modafinil, 107–108, 114t
Pyrazolopyrimidine derivative
  (zaleplon), 83–84
Pyrrolopyrazine derivative of
  cyclopyrrolone class
  (eszoplicone), 85–86

Q
QTc prolongation, from
  ziprasidone, 17–18, 18f
Quetiapine, 15–16
Quinolinone (aripiprazole),
  21–22

R
Ramelteon, 87–88
Rapid cycles, 55
Razadyne (galantamine),
  135–136
(-)-(R)-1-[4,4-Bis(3-methyl-2-
  thienyl)-3-butenyl]
  nipecotic acid hydrochloride
  (tiagabine), 67
Remeron (mirtazapine), 47–48
Revia (naltrexone), 116–117
Risperdal Consta (risperidone),
  9–10
Risperdal (risperidone), 9–10
Risperidone, 9–10
Ritalin (methylphenidate HCl),
  93–94, 113t. *See also*
  Methylphenidate (HCl)
Rivastigmine, 133–134
Rozerem (ramelteon), 87–88

S
S-3-(aminomethyl)-5-
  methylhexanoic acid
  (pregabalin), 79
(1S-cis)-4-(3,4-dichlorophenyl)-
  1,2,3,4-tetrahydro-N-
  methyl-1-nanphthal-
  enamine hydrochloride
  (sertraline), 31–32
(2S)-2,6-diamino-N-[(1S)-1-
  methyl-2-
  phenylethyl]hexanamide

dimethanesulfonate
  (lisdexamfetamine
  dimesylate), 111–112, 113t,
  115
Sedative-hypnotics, 73–88.
  See also Anxiolytics/
  sedative-hypnotics
Selegiline TS, 23–26, 24t.
  See also Antidepressants,
  first-generation
Serentil (mesoridazine), 3t
Seroquel (quetiapine), 15–16
Seroquel XR (quetiapine),
  15–16
Sertraline, 31–32
Side effects. *See also specific*
  drugs
  pediatric checklist for, 147–150
Sinequan (doxepin), 23–26, 24t.
  See also Antidepressants,
  first-generation
Sodium valproate, 57–58
Sonata (zaleplon), 83–84
Stelazine (trifluoperazine), 3t
Sterotypy, AIMS-M3D for,
  145–146
Strattera (atomoxetine),
  109–110, 114t
Substance use disorder therapy,
  116–130
  acamprosate, 127–128
  buprenorphine, 123–124
  disulfiram, 125–126
  methadone, 121–122
  naltrexone, 116–117
  naltrexone extended release,
    119–120
  varenicline, 129–130
Sulfamate-substituted
  monosaccharide
  (topiramate), 69
Sulfonamide (zonisamide), 71–72
Surmontil (trimipramine),
  23–26, 24t. *See also*
  Antidepressants, first-
  generation
Symbyax, 154–155

T
Tegretol (carbamazepine), 61–62
Temazepam (benzodiazepines),
  73–75, 74t, 75t
Tenex (guanfacine), 91–92
Thebaine derivative
  (buprenorphine), 123–124

Thieneobenzodiazepine
(olanzapine), 13–14
Thiophenepropanamine
hydrochloride (duloxetine),
51–52
Thioridazine, 2t
Thiothixene, 4t
Thorazine (chlorpromazine), 2t
Tiagabine, 67
Tic, AIMS-M3D for, 145–146
Tofranil (imipramine), 23–26,
24t. *See also*
Antidepressants,
first-generation
Topamax (topiramate), 69
Topiramate, 69
Tranylcypromine, 23–26, 24t.
See also Antidepressants,
first-generation
Trazodone, 23–26, 24t, 45–46.
See also Antidepressants,
first-generation;
Antidepressants, second-
generation
Trazolopyridine derivative
(trazodone), 23–26, 24t,
45–46. *See also*
Antidepressants, first-
generation;
Antidepressants,
second-generation
Tremor, AIMS-M3D for, 145–146
Tricyclic indan derivative
(ramelteon), 87–88

Trifluoperazine, 3t
Trilafon (perphenazine), 4t
Trileptal (oxcarbazepine),
63–64
Trimipramine, 23–26, 24t.
See also Antidepressants,
first-generation

V
Valproate, 57–58
Valproic acid (valproate), 57–58
Varenicline, 129–130
Venlafaxine, 41–42
Vivactil (protriptyline), 23–26,
24t. *See also*
Antidepressants, first-
generation
Vivitrol (naltrexone extended
release), 119–120
Vyvanse (lisdexamfetamine
dimesylate), 111–112, 113t,
115

W
Wellbutrin (bupropion), 49–50

Z
Zaleplon, 83–84
Ziprasidone, 17–19, 18f
Zoloft (sertraline), 31–32
Zolpidem, 81–82
Zonegran (zonisamide), 71–72
Zonisamide, 71–72
Zyprexa (olanzapine), 13–14